Introduction to Research Methodology for Specialist Trainees

Second edition

Introduction to Research Methodology

for

Specialist Trainees

Second edition

Edited by
P M Shaughn O'Brien and
Fiona Broughton Pipkin

ISBN 978-1-904752-01-2

Published by the **RCOG Press** at the
Royal College of Obstetricians and Gynaecologists
27 Sussex Place, Regent's Park
London NW1 4RG

Registered Charity No. 213280
RCOG Press Editor: Jane Moody
Index: Jill Halliday
Design & typesetting: Saxon Graphics Ltd, Derby
Printed by Bell and Bain Ltd, 303 Burnfield Road, Thornliebank, Glasgow G46 7UQ, UK

Contents

CONTRIBUTORS TO THE SECOND EDITION   vii

PREFACE   xi

1   Research and the specialist registrar   1
PM Shaughn O'Brien and M Fidelma O'Mahony

2   Time management   8
Charles WE Redman

3   Basic computer skills, word processing, databases, spreadsheets and presentation packages   14
Robin Burr and Andrew Welsh

4   Effective literature searching   30
Lucy Reid and Elaine Garrett

5   Critical appraisal of the research literature   58
Trish Greenhalgh

6   Evidence-based medicine and getting research into practice   69
Cindy M Farquhar

7   Audit   83
Gillian C Penney

8   Clinical trials   96
Siladitya Bhattacharya and Ashalatha Shetty

9   Animal research   113
Fiona Broughton Pipkin

10   Fetal research   121
Nicholas M Fisk and Keelin O'Donoghue

11   Laboratory research and quality control   135
D Stephen Charnock-Jones

12   Data management   141
Kirstie McKenzie-McHarg and Sarah Ayers

13   Statistics   149
Peter Brocklehurst and Simon Gates

14	Epidemiology *Paul B Silcocks*	162
15	Ethics, ethics committees, consent, fraud *Richard Kerr-Wilson*	193
16	Informing patients about research *S Andrew Spencer and Angus Dawson*	206
17	Supervising and being supervised *David M Luesley*	213
18	Applying for a grant *Katrina M Wyatt and Paul W Dimmock*	221
19	Communicating research: working with the media *David A Grimes*	230
20	Presenting a paper *Andrew Hextall and Linda Cardozo*	238
21	How to set about writing your first paper *Philip N Baker*	245
22	How to write a thesis *Jennifer Byrom*	252
	INDEX	258

Contributors to the second edition

Dr Sarah Ayers
Researcher, National Perinatal
Epidemiology Unit, Radcliffe
Infirmary, Woodstock Road,
Oxford OX2 6HE, UK

**Professor Philip N Baker
MRCOG**
Professor of Obstetrics and
Gynaecology, University of
Nottingham, Maternal and Fetal
Health Research Centre, Saint
Mary's Hospital, Whitworth Park,
Manchester M13 0JH

**Professor Siladitya Bhattacharya
FRCOG**
Consultant Obstetrician and
Gynaecologist, Aberdeen Maternity
Hospital, Cornhill Road, Aberdeen
AB25 2ZD, UK

**Dr Peter Brocklehurst MSc (Epid)
FRCOG**
Director, National Perinatal
Epidemiology Unit, Radcliffe
Infirmary, Woodstock Road,
Oxford OX2 6HE, UK

**Professor Fiona Broughton Pipkin
FRCOG**
Professor of Perinatal Physiology,
University of Nottingham, Faculty
of Medicine and Health Sciences,
Division of Obstetrics, East Block,
Queen's Medical Centre,
Nottingham NG7 2UH, UK

Dr Robin Burr MRCOG
Consultant Obstetrician and
Gynaecologist, Pontefract General
Infirmary, Friarwood Lane,
Pontefract WF8 1PL, UK

Dr Jennifer Byrom MRCOG
Clinical Assistant, Department of
Colposcopy, Birmingham Women's
Hospital, Metchley Park Road,
Edgbaston, Birmingham B15 2TG,
UK

Professor Linda Cardozo FRCOG
Professor of Urogynaecology,
King's College Hospital, Denmark
Hill, London SE5 9RS, UK

Dr D Stephen Charnock-Jones
Lecturer, University of Cambridge,
Department of Obstetrics and
Gynaecology, The Rosie Hospital,
Robinson Way, Cambridge
CB2 2SW, UK

Dr Angus Dawson
Centre for Professional Ethics,
Keele Hall, Keele University, Keele
ST5 5BG, UK

Dr Paul W Dimmock
Clinical Coordinator, School of
Medical Education, Duncan
Building, Daulby Street, Liverpool
L69 3GA, UK

Professor Cindy M Farquhar MRCOG
Postgraduate Professor of Obstetrics and Gynaecology, Department of Obstetrics and Gynaecology, National Women's Health at Auckland City Hospital, University of Auckland, Private Bag 92019, Auckland, New Zealand

Professor Nicholas M Fisk PhD FRCOG FRANZCOG DDU
Institute of Reproductive and Developmental Biology, Imperial College London, Hammersmith Campus, Du Cane Road, London W12 0NN, UK

Ms Elaine Garrett
Assistant Librarian, Royal College of Obstetricians and Gynaecologists, 27 Sussex Place, Regent's Park, London NW1 4RG, UK

Dr Simon Gates
Principal Research Fellow, Warwick Emergency Care and Rehabilitation/Warwick Clinical Trials Unit, Medical School Building, Gibbet Hill Campus, University of Warwick, Room A-101, Coventry CV4 7AL, UK

Professor Trish Greenhalgh
Department of Primary Care and Population Sciences, Royal Free and University College Medical School, Holborn Union Building, Archway Campus, Highgate Hill, London N19 5NF, UK

Professor David A Grimes
Clinical Professor, Department of Obstetrics and Gynaecology, University of North Carolina School of Medicine, Chapel Hill, North Carolina 27514, USA and Vice President of Biomedical Affairs, Family Health International, PO Box 13950, Research Triangle Park, North Carolina 27709, USA

Mr Andrew Hextall MD MRCOG
Consultant Obstetrician and Gynaecologist, Women's Services Directorate, St Albans City Hospital, Waverley Road, St Albans AL3 5PN, UK

Mr Richard Kerr-Wilson FRCOG
Consultant Obstetrician and Gynaecologist, Cheltenham General Hospital, Sandford Road, Cheltenham, Gloucester GL53 7AN, UK

Professor David M Luesley FRCOG
Professor of Gynaecological Oncology, Academic Department of Gynaecological Oncology, Birmingham Women's Hospital, Metchley Park Road, Birmingham B15 2TG, UK

Dr Kirstie McKenzie-McHarg
Trials Coordinator/Researcher, National Perinatal Epidemiology Unit, Radcliffe Infirmary, Woodstock Road, Oxford OX2 6HE, UK

Professor PM Shaughn O'Brien
Professor and Head of Academic
Department of Obstetrics and
Gynaecology, North Staffordshire
Hospital, Maternity Unit, City
General Hospital, Newcastle Road,
Stoke-on-Trent ST4 6QG, UK

**Dr Keelin O'Donoghue PhD
MRCOG**
Subspecialty Trainee in Maternal
and Fetal Medicine and Honorary
Clinical Lecturer, Imperial College
London, Centre for Fetal Care,
Queen Charlotte's and Chelsea
Hospital, Du Cane Road, London
W12 0HS, UK

Miss Fidelma O'Mahony
Senior Lecturer in Medical
Education/Consultant in Obstetrics
and Gynaecology, University
Hospital of North Staffordshire,
Newcastle Road, Stoke-on-Trent
ST4 6QG, UK

**Dr Gillian C Penney MD FRCOG
MFFP**
National Coordinator, Scottish
Programme for Clinical Effectiveness
in Reproductive Health, Dugald
Baird Centre for Research on
Women's Health, Aberdeen
Maternity Hospital, Cornhill Road,
Aberdeen AB25 2ZL, UK

Mr Charles WE Redman FRCOG
Consultant Obstetrician and
Gynaecologist, Academic
Department of Obstetrics and
Gynaecology, North Staffordshire
Hospital, Maternity Unit, City
General Hospital, Newcastle Road,
Stoke-on-Trent ST4 6QG, UK

Ms Lucy Reid
Head of Information Services,
Royal College of Obstetricians and
Gynaecologists, 27 Sussex Place,
Regent's Park, London NW1 4RG,
UK

Dr Ashalatha Shetty MRCOG
Clinical Research Fellow, Assisted
Reproduction Unit, Aberdeen
Maternity Hospital, Cornhill Road,
Aberdeen AB25 2ZD, UK

Dr Paul B Silcocks
Associate Director, Research and
Development, Trent Cancer
Registry, Weston Park Hospital
NHS Trust, Whitham Road,
Sheffield S10 2SJ, UK

Dr S Andrew Spencer
Honorary Consultant Paediatrician,
Reader in Neonatal Medicine, Keele
University, Neonatal Unit, City
General Hospital, Newcastle Road,
Stoke-on-Trent ST4 6QG, UK

Dr Katrina M Wyatt
Lecturer in Health Services
Research, Exeter & North Devon
Research & Development Support
Unit, Noy Scott House, Haldon
View Terrace, Exeter EX2 5EQ,
UK

Mr Andrew Welsh
Advanced Member, Society for
Editors and Proofreaders, Flat 4, 30
Clyde Road, Croydon CR0 6SU,
UK

Preface

Professor Broughton Pipkin and I have written and published together inter-mittently over the past 30 years, particularly in the early part of this time when we were both with the Academic Department of Obstetrics and Gynaecology at the City Hospital, Nottingham. In that time medical research has seen many changes. The role, place and even the purpose of undertaking research has changed.

This text is written for trainees – not just medical trainees but trainees in all subjects related to health. Because of the nature of our posts and contacts there is a resulting emphasis on the specialist registrar trainee and many of the writers and thus the examples in the text are obstetric and gynaecological – physicians and surgeons need not feel threatened by this!

It is also true that research questions will creep into Royal College mem-bership examinations over the next couple of years.

Whether it is the spirit of enquiry, the pursuit of an original idea or prag-matism of obtaining Membership of your College or a research degree to enable your ascent up one of the many career ladders, we hope that this text provides encouragement, insight and direction.

Fiona Broughton Pipkin
Shaughn O'Brien

1

Research and the specialist registrar

PM Shaughn O'Brien and M Fidelma O'Mahony

Why do research?

Specialist registrar (SpR) training is now well established and, along with it, the need to develop an understanding of research methodology. There are, however, many motives for undertaking research. These include the (fairly remote) chance of making an important discovery, the enjoyment of the process of undertaking research, the hope of altering accepted management of a disease and making patients better through your own discovery and there is the buzz of working in an intellectual environment. You will note that financial reward does not appear in this list, for very good reasons. Only a few researchers (and no SpRs) have yet received a Nobel Prize.

There are other reasons for undertaking research which are more pragmatic. There are questions on research methodology in Membership examinations of the Royal Colleges. The Government is increasing clinical and translational research. Academic medicine and, more precisely, research provides the basic evidence for the provision of health care, together with advances in molecular and cell biology and medicine, reproductive medicine, imaging, pharmaceutical and hormonal advances, advances in surgery, which all provide the platform for research at all levels including training. Furthermore, formal research is now a requirement in all subspecialty training programmes. On completion of training, it is usually easier to obtain a consultant post with an MD ('awarded' not 'in preparation') and those who have demonstrated their ability to be 'doers' and 'completer/finishers' will be rewarded with a greater choice of consultant posts when the time comes. It is rare to be appointed even to non-academic posts in teaching hospitals or other major centres without a higher degree in addition to Membership of a Royal College. Few consultants are now appointed to their first choice of post without having, at the very least, published some peer-reviewed papers.

But what of the gap between obtaining the membership and the much sought after training number and finally obtaining the elusive consultant post? Research is now more important than ever in honing the subtle yet essential skills of presentation, of both oneself and one's work. Trainees may now arrive at their consultant interview with relatively little experience in 'selling themselves', thanks to the introduction of structured training. The benefits of undertaking research extend far beyond the interview process as it is increasingly recognised that achieving a consultant post no longer marks the end of training.

Carrying out a research project and presenting their work to an audience has several educational advantages for the SpR. It fosters an independent and questioning thought process, as well as the ability to communicate effectively. Lifelong learning demands that professionals remain conversant with current developments. In addition, we cannot ignore the forward march of information technology whereby our patients have almost equal access to research information, and often approach the consultation brandishing what amounts to a literature search! No one can be expected to deal with this without having first-hand experience of research themselves. Of course, any trainee wishing ultimately to pursue a career in academic medicine will need to obtain a postgraduate research degree such as an MD or, increasingly, a PhD.

Training programmes have, however, changed significantly in recent years, with the development of the Foundation programme (F1, F2), followed by the new run-through grade of specialist training leading to the award of the Certificate of Completion of Training (CCT). The recommendations of the 1993 report, *Hospital Doctors: Training for the Future*[1] (the Calman Report) clearly stated that those responsible, at government level, for defining the training of hospital specialists were aware of the needs and opportunities for research during specialist training. It was recommended that all doctors in training should learn how to interpret and apply research findings and that specific provision should be made for those who wish to undertake research and/or prepare for an academic career.

The UK Clinical Research Collaboration (UKCRC) is a partnership of organisations working to establish the UK as a world leader in clinical research, by harnessing the power of the NHS. Its aim is to re-engineer the environment in which clinical research is conducted in the UK, to benefit the public and patients by improving national health and increasing national wealth, Much of which will be achieved in collaboration with the Royal College of Obstetricians and Gynaecologists (RCOG) and other Royal Colleges.

In 2005, the Academic Careers Sub-committee of Modernising Medical Careers and the UK Clinical Research Collaboration laid out plans for incorporating this principle into the new career structure.[2] This provides structure for academic clinical fellowships and lecturer posts for which trainees may apply.

The basic principle of the SpR grade is that, during their specialist training, doctors should be expected to develop an understanding of research methodology (and this is why the MRCOG examination increasingly includes questions related to audit, research papers, assessment of clinical trials and the interpretation of data) and should be encouraged to undertake research.

There are four main groups of doctors who will wish to undertake research during higher specialist training:

- The majority of doctors who undertake a period in research during higher specialist training will ultimately wish to pursue a clinical career. They will aim to complete a specialist training programme and to be awarded a Certificate of Completion of Training (CCT) giving them access to the Specialist Register. Good peer-reviewed papers may be as appropriate as a research degree for this group. A smaller group of doctors who intend to pursue a career in academic or research medicine will, in most cases, also wish to obtain a CCT in a recognised discipline. Although these doctors should have no less thorough clinical training than other SpRs, the content of their training programme, while meeting the requirements set out in the appropriate College curriculum, will have to take into account the need to develop both their research and their clinical skills. Academic career pathways will be both attractive and flexible in all respects. Academic career structures will ensure that both clinical and academic training are appropriate. Many will be linked to subspecialty training posts but not all. Specific posts will be designated as National Training Number (Academic) – NTN(A). The aim is to produce academic clinicians of the highest calibre. Note that the RCOG (the first college to do so) has devised the new academic curriculum, which has been approved by the Postgraduate Medical Education and Training Board.
- While development of educational skills will also be an important component of training, education in itself is now well established as a separate career research choice. It has already been made clear in the report published by Lord Dearing that the acquisition of 'key skills' related to learning and imparting knowledge should still be a formal goal even at doctoral level.
- All subspecialty training programmes involve an important research component. It is often difficult to obtain such training posts without having undertaken research, usually to the level of MD. It is a mandatory component of the subspecialty training programme to have produced either a research thesis or to have published two first-author papers in citable refereed journals before the subspecialty recognition of the CCT can be awarded. These trainees may ultimately become pure clinical subspecialists or academics.
- A very small group of trainees may ultimately go into highly specialised fields of predominantly research work and very little clinical work.

What should be my research aims?

The individual's purpose in undertaking the research will dictate when and how it is undertaken. The goal will thus vary but publication in one way or another is essential. If research has been performed but not published then it is considered incomplete and better if not started in the first place. This is because of the waste of the researcher's and collaborator's/supervisor's time and the waste of resources. The ethics of patient-based research that is subsequently not published is high on the agenda. There are many ways in which research can be published:

- as a verbal presentation or poster with a published abstract (this should normally be followed by a full publication)
- as a peer-reviewed research paper
- as a higher degree thesis
- as a part of a review article
- as an electronic publication (for example, *The Cochrane Library*).

All undergraduates should have been introduced to research at an early stage when producing a dissertation or mini-thesis in part fulfilment of the requirements for a degree. A dissertation may form part of a:

- Bachelor of Science (BSc) degree
- Master of Science (MSc)
- Bachelor of Medical Science (BMedSci)
- Master of Medical Science (MMed Sci)
- Master of Philosophy (MPhil)
- Doctor of Philosophy (PhD)
- Doctor of Medicine (MD)
- Doctor of Surgery (MCh)
- Doctor of Science (DSc).

The BSc, MSc and BMedSci degrees are usually taught, with a dissertation providing a proportion of the credits. MPhil is usually a research-based degree by thesis and most universities require the candidate to register for this before being 'promoted' to PhD on the basis of progress of the research and the researcher.

The PhD has previously been considered to be more scientifically oriented and the MD more clinically based research, although there is much overlap these days. PhD theses have always been closely supervised, while MD theses were not until recently. There are historical grounds for this. Until relatively recently, the MD tended to be more of a distillation of many years of clinical research experience focused on a particular topic, rather than a structured investigation. This has changed. All research theses are now considered as research training and all are formally supervised, which is appropriate. A DSc, in most universities, is awarded following the submission of work and many research papers that represent a sustained contribution to medical knowledge by a recognised authority in a particular field of medicine or science.

In general, research undertaken by non-medical graduates would be as part of an MPhil or PhD and usually requires 3–4 years of single-minded study for completion. Medical specialist trainees would do a PhD or MD. A PhD is more internationally accepted as a research higher degree and those aspiring to an academic career at a high level would, in the present day, perhaps be well advised to pursue this line. Furthermore, in the USA and in parts of Asia and the Middle East, the MD is the name of the basic medical degree, which can give rise to confusion. The MD can be and often is completed in 2 years, the PhD usually takes 3 years.

The MMedSci degree is a developing degree particularly suited to the non-subspecialist trainee. These degrees usually contain a considerable taught element, including such subjects as ethics, law, epidemiology, theoretical research methodology, statistics, medical education, clinical effectiveness, science and technology or health service management.

In addition, there are specialty-specific training modules which may also be recognised for other training (but, of course, not for another degree). Examples would include recognised laparoscopic surgery training, ultrasound/imaging and so on. Finally, there is a specialty-related research dissertation and this is what usually distinguishes a Masters degree from a Diploma. This type of degree may eventually prove to be more appropriate than an MD for the non-academic trainee, in that it provides the foundation for those skills and knowledge required by the consultant of the future. The supervised research within this would be more than adequate to provide an understanding of research methodology as required by the time of attainment of the CCT.

What subject should you research?

The content and conduct of your research is, in theory, down to personal choice. However, it is rarely that simple. Funding must be provided for salaries and the expenses of equipment and material. It is virtually impossible to make a successful research application without research experience and a track record. In other words, you will be dependent on the support of an established researcher or research unit. You will need a great deal of training and supervision from the outset and so the only practical way forward is to apply for a post in an established unit which will provide all of these. These posts will almost invariably be externally funded by a grant awarding body or using 'soft' (grant) money. It takes time, perseverance and luck to obtain such money. Start planning early with your potential supervisor.

The range of research open to SpRs is enormous. It can be in clinical trials, laboratory research, basic science, epidemiology, social science, psychology, biomedical engineering and technology, imaging, screening, education, molecular medicine and so on and these can be conducted in animal research, hospital or general practice patients, healthy volunteers, computer models or indeed in libraries. There are also recognised clinical research training fellowships, such as those, for example, from the Medical Research Council (MRC) and the Wellcome Trust.

An increasing number of research units recognise detailed literature reviews and meta-analyses as fully adequate for a research thesis. Many others would think that such research is merely the starting point for genuine research. An initial literature review is always necessary to determine that an important question remains unanswered and that your new trial or study is justified from an economic (time and money) and ethical standpoint.

When should I undertake research during training?

There is a risk that Calman training, shortening of training, the new run-through grade and the need to produce consultants rapidly will be a threat to SpR research. Academic medicine is under threat through a combination of under funding and under recruitment. Modernising Medical Careers is addressing this by developing academic foundation programmes. Having completed this, a successful candidate will then apply for an NTN(A). The Government has introduced the requirement for a basic understanding of research and enquiry into secondary school education at Key Stage 3 of the National Curriculum. All undergraduates should be introduced to research at an early stage. All current training in health subjects addresses research in the course of training and all medical schools allow undergraduates to take a research-based intercalated BSc degree, usually taken by those identified as 'high flyers'. In addition, in *Tomorrow's Doctors*[3] the General Medical Council clearly states that 25–30% of the undergraduate curriculum should comprise of student selected components (SSC). In this period, students are encouraged to undertake a research project in an area of their choosing.

The arrangements for specialist training have, at least in theory, been designed to be as flexible as possible for doctors wishing to pursue many career pathways. It is essential therefore that those following a purely clinical career have the opportunity to develop the research know-how to interpret research data and use this in their decision making when they treat patients, while those wishing to follow an academic career attain the desired clinical competencies to undertake their clinical work and achieve the CCT. Others will wish to follow a career which is predominantly academic, with a balance of clinical work, teaching and research. A very small group will become so taken by their research that they abandon clinical work altogether in favour of a career as a clinical scientist.

A further consideration is the changing demographics of medicine. The majority of medical school applicants are female and the Royal Colleges and the Academic Careers Sub-committee of Modernising Medical Careers and the UK Clinical Research Collaboration have recognised this in their work-force planning. Flexibility within clinical and academic careers is now an acknowledged necessity. This extends beyond working hours planning to include choice in point of entry to training programmes allowing for career breaks. This system is to be supported by a comprehensive mentorship scheme providing trainees with practical and pastoral support. You will probably not know to which of the preceding categories you belong. You cannot really know until you are well into your research training. The contribution of all of these people is vital to the future of individual specialties and indeed to the NHS.

The chapters which follow in this book deal with many of the subjects above, and more, in great detail. They will provide valuable support for the novice and a source of inspiration for budding academics and thinking clinicians.

References

1. Calman K. *Hospital doctors: training for the future.* (Dd DH 004113 4/93) London: HMSO; 1993.
2. UK Clinical Research Collaboration. *Report of the Academic Careers Sub-Committee of Modernising Medical Careers and the Clinical Research Collaboration Medically and Dentally-qualified Academic Staff: Recommendations for training the researchers and educators of the future.* London: UKCRC; 2005 [www.ukcrc.org].
3. General Medical Council. *Tomorrow's Doctors.* London: GMC; 2003.

Further reading

BMJ *Career Focus* 2002;325:7354.
British Medical Association. *Women in Academic Medicine: Challenges and issues. A report by Health Policy and Economic Research Unit.* London: BMA; 2004.
UK Clinical Research Collaboration, Department of Health. *New Academic Training Pathways for Medical and Dental Graduates: A Pocket Guide.* London: DH; 2005.

2

Time management

Charles WE Redman

Introduction

Involvement in research, whether as a research fellow or in a clinical post, provides the opportunity of learning a variety of different skills and disciplines. Many of these will have a wider application in your clinical career and none more so than time management. Time is said to be a linear parameter but during research its passage can defy physics. At first it may stretch out into the future almost infinitely and pass so slowly that the challenge is how to fill it. Then, ever faster, as in free-fall skydiving, the deadlines rush towards you. The key to success, be it in research or in a medical career generally, is to manage time. A number of excellent texts describe classic time management but to save your time, this short chapter summarises their key points.

'Doing' is not necessarily achieving and this is particularly so in research. 'Research is to see what everybody else has seen, and to think what nobody else has thought' (Albert Szent-Györgyi, discoverer of vitamin C and Nobel Prize winner). Thinking needs time which has to be set aside, not only for thought but also for planning.

Planning

At the outset of any project or task there are three key questions that you need to address. These are:
- How much time do I have?
- What do I have to do?
- How am I going to do it?

The first question is usually the easiest as this is often defined for you either in terms of funding or stated deadlines. It can relate to a longer period, such as the duration of a research fellowship, or simply to the forthcoming week or day. It is important to have determined at the outset how much time is to be spent working rather than in other important areas of your life. It is also prudent to make your plans with time to spare, as there are inevitably interruptions or unscheduled hitches that would otherwise compromise your plans. In short, be realistic and not over-ambitious.

The second question is not so straightforward, as there are often supplementary ones such as whether you need or should be doing it anyway. But if this is something you need to do then it becomes a 'goal'. At any one time you may have a number of goals and the process for achieving them can be broken down into smaller, individual, tasks. The third item is about realising these tasks within the timescale you have set and requires drawing up a timetable.

Setting goals

A goal defines what you want to achieve, be it in life generally or professionally. In the context of research it can be obtaining a thesis, a grant, a publication or whatever it is you are wanting as the return for your investment of time and effort.

If you are taking a long-term strategic view, such as 'What do I want in life?' or 'What am I aiming to achieve in the next 2 years?', you will identify a number of major goals which you then work towards. To this end you will probably identify a number of minor goals to aim for on the way, as you move towards your major goal. Clearly there are different orders of goals depending on the time frame in which you are working. In other words, as you write your thesis, a major goal, you need to have the introduction written by next month, a minor goal.

You will usually have a number of different goals which are all making demands on your time and often threatening to outstrip it. It is unrealistic to have too many major goals, as you will be at risk of fighting on too many fronts and winning nothing. So it is also vital that before you launch into the fray you have decided which goals are the most important and planned accordingly.

In practical terms it is a good idea to sit down every so often to review what your goals are and how you are progressing. This may be every year, or more often, but you must have in mind your priorities as this will determine how you spend your time.

Tasking

The individual steps towards reaching goals are tasks. The relationship between major goals, minor goals and tasks is hierarchical and is best illustrated by the tree analogy (Figure 2.1) in which the trunk equals the major goal, the branches are the minor goals and the leaves are tasks.

The key point about this concept is that large pieces of work can be broken down into smaller manageable parts. People are often daunted by the size of

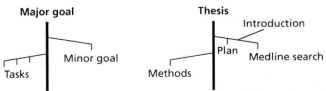

Figure 2.1 The relationship between major goals, minor goals and tasks

certain projects, but this can be overcome by breaking them down into their component parts. In other words:

Q: How do you eat an elephant?

A: In many meals and in little pieces!

Prioritisation

Having defined your goals and identified the component tasks that are going to need to be achieved within a given time, say the next week, you will have a list of items all competing for your time. If it is unlikely that you will be able to do all these tasks, you will have to decide what to do, what not to do and what you may do if there is time. This is prioritisation.

One method is to triage the tasks into one of three categories, namely:

- essential
- important
- less important.

That bit is easy but it is how you do it that counts. It could be done purely on the basis of deadlines or whether the tasks are important to you, to others or to no one in particular. Whatever method you use, the important thing is that the jobs to do are prioritised so that the important tasks get done, even if this has to be at the expense of less important ones. If you do not prioritise the reverse often happens.

This exercise is worth doing on a weekly basis as you work out what needs doing in the time available. Make a list of what has to be done and prioritise each task. Having made this list, it can be helpful to rewrite the list using a column for each priority (Figure 2.2). Produce your timetable of available time and allocate time to each task in order of priority. If you run out of available time, so be it. If you do not have enough time to achieve the top priority tasks then you have a problem. Either your prior planning has been poor or you have an unrealistic number of major goals and something has to go. If the balloon is sinking you have to throw something out.

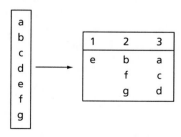

Figure 2.2 Prioritise goals and tasks. Make a list of the tasks to do and then sort them into priority categories

Timetabling

Much of the above is about timetabling but it is worth making some additional points. Firstly, be realistic about how long something will take. It is counterproductive to produce an over-ambitious plan for the week and doom yourself to failure at the outset. In addition, be realistic about what should be done in the time available; do not try making a silk purse out of a sow's ear and do what you can. Stop doing it when it is good enough. It is pointless striving for perfection and going well down the path of diminishing returns when that time could have been better used for something else.

When making out your timetable leave enough time to eat, sleep, relax and enjoy yourself. Furthermore, if at any stage you achieve targets ahead of schedule, do not necessarily rush on to the next one but take advantage of this lull to reward yourself with a break and do something different.

Deadlines

Much of time management is about working to deadlines. In research, most deadlines concern dates of submission for grants or abstracts when plenty of notice is available. The cardinal rule about deadlines is that you should not break them and should do everything in your power to meet them. If others set the deadline, you have to decide at the outset whether the task is worth doing and if the deadline is reasonable. There is no point in committing yourself to something that cannot be done in the time available; instead, you should decline it or renegotiate the deadline. To do otherwise compounds the felony and only puts your head on the block. However, once you have accepted a deadline, be it set by yourself or others, you must work to it.

Saving time

While planning is an essential part of making the best use of time, working efficiently is also important. There are a number of skills that can help significantly. Learn to say 'No' and avoid doing somebody else's work. Wherever possible delegate tasks to others but do so appropriately as failure will rebound on you. Master information technology skills, including how to type. Direct input of data into computer spreadsheets or databases is a vital skill and, increasingly, a laptop is essential. Nonetheless, despite the acquisition of these other skills, planning remains pivotal. Without planning, your work will be entropic. One example of the efficient use of time is, in the course of presenting your work at meetings, to work on the relevant papers at this time. It is much easier to do this while the ideas and responses of other participants are fresh in your mind. All too often work is presented and the paper is written much later.

Wasting time

'I would I could stand at a busy corner, hat in hand, and beg people to throw me all their wasted hours' (Bernard Berenson). Whatever gains you make by working more efficiently can be dissipated by the time you waste. It is sometimes worth making a log of how you spend your time, so you can analyse how it is actually spent. This can help you to identify those tasks that you could have avoided or delegated to others, as well as suggest ways in which you could work better. Why go to the library on three separate occasions when you could have done what you wanted to do in a single visit?

One of the greatest hindrances to getting things done is procrastination. This often occurs because the task in question is seen as large and daunting while other smaller, but less important, tasks can be easily done in the time available. You must avoid this. Breaking the larger tasks down into smaller parts which can be tackled in the time available is the key.

Delegation

This is a potentially important way of saving time. When facing a task it is advised that you should decide if (a) it needs doing and (b) should you be doing it? Whenever possible avoid carrying out a task that could or should be carried out by someone else; this can be done in one of three ways:

- refusal
- palming off
- delegation.

If you have no vested interest in the task and it is not your responsibility, then simply say 'No'. However, it may be easier to 'palm off' the task to someone else. The difference between this and delegation is that when you palm off a task you are indifferent to the outcome, whereas when you delegate you care. In other words, although delegation can save time, you retain responsibility. Consequently, it is in your best interests to ensure that your delegation is carried out appropriately; that is, the right task for the right person with adequate explanation and supervision. Poor delegation will result in your having to undo what has been done, or doing the job yourself, and be counterproductive. It is important to recognise that, initially, delegation may be a time-consuming activity as you ensure that things are done properly. The saying 'if you want a job doing properly, do it yourself' is not necessarily the case when delegation works. Incentives, such as co-authorship or acknowledgement, promote successful delegation and failure to give due recognition will jeopardise future success.

Delegation implies the handing-down of a task, whereas most junior researchers are already in the basement. However, there is often scope for collaboration in which tasks can be shared. Indeed, an increasing feature of modern clinical research is the formation of teams comprising individuals providing different skills, such as clinicians, biochemists, statisticians, data managers. Nonetheless, whether you delegate or collaborate, the process has to be thought through and not simply be allowed to happen, lest it become counterproductive.

Hiding

There are many detractors from study:

- bleeps
- supervisors
- NHS colleagues saying 'We're short, come and help out with the clinic'
- patients
- colleagues, friends and family.

One way of ring-fencing your time is to identify a location which is protected from the outside world. This could be a study, a carrel in the library, a train or an aeroplane.

Final comments

Time spent in research can be very rewarding, providing the opportunity to learn a variety of skills which often have wider application. The time available for research is limited for most doctors and it is a precious resource which to some degree can be expanded or lost depending on its use. 'Gather ye rose-buds while ye may, Old Time is still a-flying' (Robert Herrick, 1591–1674, *To the Virgins, to Make Much of Time*).

3

Basic computer skills, word processing, databases, spreadsheets and presentation packages

Robin Burr and Andrew Welsh

The advent of the electronic age has revolutionised the way we work and communicate. The rapid and continuing advances in this technology have given the individual user the type of processing power in a personal computer (PC) that previously was only available in large mainframe machines. The PC has provided the scientific worker and clinician with an invaluable tool for their work. Not only have previously laborious work practices been transformed but the PC has enabled entirely new ways of working to be developed. Possibly the most useful advance for the research worker is the electronic transfer of information between computers, both locally and globally over the internet. The fierce competition in the PC market has ensured that a relatively powerful combination of hardware and software is an inexpensive option that all researchers should be using to enhance the quality of their efforts. This chapter is intentionally basic; most advances beyond this will be best obtained from practical experience, together with informal advice from more experienced users or courses run by the university.

Basic computing skills

In the days of DOS (disk operating system), from 1981 until the early 1990s, the PC user had to learn a complex series of commands to operate the computer, followed by another set of commands for each application program used. Every program would itself have its own individual set of commands which would often be very different from any other program with similar functions. These commands would have to be typed in at a command line with reference to a bulky manual. Thankfully for those of us with limited keyboard skills but reasonable hand–eye coordination, the advent of the Microsoft Windows® operating system, especially from version 3.1 in 1992, provided a graphical interface together with a mouse (a pointing device controlling an on-screen cursor and other functions) to provide a simpler means of interacting with the computer. On-screen help became available and the manuals started becoming thinner. However, there were still large differences in the way in which the various application programs interfaced with the user, with very few being intuitive.

As Windows is the most widely used operating system in the world, this chapter will concentrate on software that runs on this operating system. When buying a new PC it will usually be preloaded with Windows XP® or Windows Vista as the operating system and will often also come with one or other of the major suites of application programs, most probably Microsoft Works or Microsoft Office.

Currently, all the mainstream software packages have comprehensive on-screen help which enables the first-time user to achieve a decent level of proficiency in a relatively short time. This online help varies from the vital to the extremely irritating, according to the level of expertise of the user, although most can be switched off. Most software manuals are quite short in content and, consequently, there is now a large market for independent books explaining how to use the main software packages. Examples include the *Que Quick Reference* series and the *For Dummies* series covering all the major software programs.

To the average individual there are no significant differences between the various software packages, in that the ability of each program is well in excess of the needs of the average user. In fact it has been estimated that, for 80% of the time, the average user only uses 20% of the functions in a software program. So the choice of which software programs to use depends on variables such as which particular software was sold with the computer or which screen appearance is preferable or which software is used at work. All the major programs will be able to read the data files created by their competitors and most provide a relatively easy means of converting other files into their own format.

Word processing

Possibly the most valuable program for the average user is the word processing program. One major advantage of the PC is that work can be stored on a disk (either a memory stick, DVD or CD-ROM) for transfer between computers or on the internal hard disk, for future amendments and editing. Any number of copies, in a variety of formats, can be printed without having to retype a single word. If amendments are necessary, these can very easily be incorporated without having to retype the whole document. The same piece of work can also be printed to a wide variety of printers. The creator has total control over the final appearance of the printed work and can easily preview a variety of different versions on-screen prior to printing the final version. In fact, the latest versions of the major word processors are so sophisticated that there is a large overlap with the functions usually found in desktop publishing programs. The major word processing packages are Microsoft's Word, IBM's Lotus Word Pro® and Corel's WordPerfect®. There are no significant differences in functionality between these programs and personal preference is the best reason for preferring one over another.

Other functions that are invaluable for producing a professional-quality document include the spellchecker, format checker and thesaurus. Although the standard spellchecker is unlikely to contain specialised and technical words, these can be added to a user dictionary or even bought as additions to the main program. The ability to create tables of contents and indexes together with the creation of graphs, tables and graphics including equations are functions available in all the major programs. All the main word processing programs now provide integration with the other programs in the suite so that graphs, spreadsheets and databases can be readily incorporated into a document with the advantage that, when the original is changed, the copy in the document is automatically updated. Mail merging is a useful function when a standard letter has to be sent to a large number of people – this is commonly seen in the vast and increasing amount of 'personalised' junk mail delivered by the postal service.

As increasing numbers of publications are now multi-authored, a fast and convenient means of reviewing the article is afforded by emailing the word processor file to all the authors either over a local area network (such as a university network) or globally via the internet. The advantage of this method of communication over posted or faxed versions is that the second author can make corrections and amendments directly to the original document, prior to emailing it back to the first author. Furthermore, the 'track changes' feature allows changes, insertions and deletions from multiple contributors to be shown. These changes can subsequently be accepted or rejected one at a time or as a whole.

For the researcher with references to organise, a reference manager program can save an enormous amount of time. Although there is no shortcut to the time-consuming chore of entering the individual references into the program, its value when formatting the final paper soon becomes apparent. For an additional expense, this type of program can also import references electronically from CD-ROM or via Medline. All these programs can produce a bibliography in a wide variety of standard formats required by the major journals in a fraction of the time it would take to do the same process manually. Should the style of the bibliography need changing, for example, for submission to another journal, this can easily be accomplished without having to retype any of the original document. Of course, the database of references created can be used for any number of documents in the future.

For those that find typing difficult and slow, there are now voice recognition programs that translate the spoken word into the typewritten version. Although attractive at first sight, there are limitations with this type of program and they still require a fair amount of typing to correct errors, even after extensive training of the program. Such programs may, however, eventually become the standard method of interfacing with a PC. In the meantime, a short course on typing skills may, for most of us, prove to be more valuable than the detailed anatomy of the mid-brain!

Databases

Although word processing is probably the most common use for a PC, their real value is in data processing. The PC is essentially a simple calculator and is ideal for processing any form of data, both numerical and text. A notebook computer provides a method of collecting data in the field and a network of PCs allows many users to enter data into the same database.

A database provides a standardised method of entering data and each data field can be validated, in that only one of a set number of responses can be entered into that field. The database can readily be updated and amendments easily made if necessary. Also, an entry for each field can be required by the program to avoid loss of data. These are both major advantages over a paper-based method of data collection. Storing data on a PC provides a compact method of storage when compared with the paper-based method, although a secure means of backing up or making a copy of the data is vital. Remember, researchers have lost whole PhD theses in computer crashes or faulty floppy disks. A 'belt and braces' approach is strongly recommended to back up all-important data, both electronically and paper-based.

The real strength of databases is evident when the collected data are then collated and processed. Performing searches on a computerised database is infinitely quicker and more accurate than hand-searching a mass of paper forms. Not only that, but complex searches can easily be created and saved for later reuse. The subset of data thus found can then be saved into a new file or imported into a spreadsheet for statistical analysis. New data fields can be created through performing calculations on existing data fields and then incorporated into searches.

Database programs may either be 'flat file' or 'relational' in nature. Flat file databases store each record as an individual item so that any field common to another record must be retyped into each and every record. This can be time consuming where there is a large amount of data common to each record such as where one patient has a number of observations made at different times – the patient details would have to be entered into each record of the observations at every event. A relational database stores the data in several separate files that are cross-referenced. In the above example the patient data would only be entered once into a separate file then cross-referenced with the observational data files as required. Although this would require slightly more time to create, it allows for a very efficient and powerful database to be developed. Each file created can be cross-referenced or linked to any other database file and can thus be reused any number of times. When considering using a database, the additional effort required in creating a relational database will provide its own rewards when using the database both to enter and, later, process the data. The latest versions of the major database programs all provide ready- made templates and help routines for creating quite complex databases without needing any knowledge of programming.

Database programs provide a number of ways of producing output. This may take the form of a printed report, a graph or a file incorporated into another document. Again, the major programs all provide a great deal of help in producing whatever type of output is required.

Designing a database is relatively easy but needs careful consideration together with a number of 'dry runs' prior to the main data entry as it can be difficult to reconfigure the database later, when it already contains a quantity of precious data. It is also important to consider the end use of data in that there is very little point in having collected a quantity of data that cannot later be processed in a useful and meaningful manner. For example, many maternity databases are easy to enter data into but have limited or no facility for the non-standard searches that a researcher would want to perform. Where there will be a need for statistical analysis of the data collected it is well worth considering the type of data output that the statistical program or a statistician will require when designing the database. Advice of this nature should be sought during the design phase of the research protocol and its database.

Spreadsheets

A spreadsheet program provides a powerful means of manipulating data, ranging from simple calculations to complex statistical and financial functions. Multiple calculations can be performed on the data set on a 'what if' basis, that is, determining the effect of changing one piece of data on the rest of the data set without losing any of the original data. This is particularly, although not exclusively, valuable in financial spreadsheets.

A spreadsheet consists of a number of cells labelled alphabetically along the columns and numerically down the rows. Each cell can contain any type of data, both numerical and text, or formulae. The major programs come with a wide and comprehensive range of formulae that include means of manipulating financial, mathematical, statistical, trigonometrical, calendar, logical and text-based data among others. Data can readily be sorted and sub-sorted in any order on any particular type of criteria, alphabetical, numerical or by date.

Spreadsheets also include database-type functions, which are particularly useful for managing small volumes of data, although for large amounts of data a specific database program is more suitable. Most spreadsheets will allow data to be imported or directly linked to data within a database, although usually only from the database within the same manufacturer's suite of programs.

All spreadsheets come with extensive and powerful charting capabilities for producing professional-quality figures, either directly from the program itself or when imported into or linked to a word processor file. A colour inkjet or laser printer will demonstrate the impressive quality of charting output from a spreadsheet program.

Statistical analysis has always been a strong point of spreadsheet programs and is usually an integral part of any research project. Depending on the nature and complexity of the analysis (and the ability of the researcher) the spreadsheet program may provide all the required functions. Even if this is all that is required for data analysis it is wise to seek the advice of a statistician prior to collecting and analysing data. For larger data sets and complex analyses a statistical package may be a better means of analysing the data. In this case, discussion with the statistician using the statistical program will ensure that not only is the correct data collected but also that the output from the spreadsheet program is compatible with the statistical program.

The most recent versions of spreadsheet programs offer what is known as '3D spreadsheets'. In this situation a number of separate spreadsheets can be interlinked such that calculations can be performed on cells across a number of different spreadsheets, with the results exported to or saved in a separate spreadsheet.

Although spreadsheets were initially the program that made the PC a valuable tool, they have had a reputation for being difficult to use. This has largely, although not entirely, been addressed by the software manufacturers, who have included a number of templates and help routines for creating new spreadsheets. Spreadsheets, columns and ranges of data can now be labelled with more intuitive names which can, in turn, be used in calculations and formulas.

Presentation packages

All researchers will have to present their work at some point, and whether this is an in-house talk or a presentation at an international meeting, good-quality visual aids are essential for getting the message across clearly. The advantage of using a PC to produce these visual aids is that the creator has total control over the content and appearance of the work. Not only that, but the original files are stored on disk and can be reused to produce any number and type of output.

The simplest and cheapest means of providing a visual aid is to photocopy the printed output from a word processor onto acetates, for use with an overhead projector. Although well-considered use of fonts and arrangement can produce a clear overhead, this method is rather limited. Use of a colour inkjet printer with the appropriate acetates will allow colour overheads to be produced directly from the PC at short notice. Virtually all auditoriums, however small, will have an overhead projector, which is relatively simple technology. Whatever the primary means of presenting, it may be worth having a (colour) copy on overheads as a backup.

A specialised presentation package will provide a more comprehensive method of producing a presentation in a number of formats. This provides total control over all aspects of producing a slide and will create a common appearance to all the slides in the presentation. A variety of graphics are provided with the program or can be imported from clip art or created with the aid of a scanner or digital camera. Most also have a comprehensive range of graphics to produce organisational and flow charts. All the programs have templates and help routines for the relatively easy creation of a presentation.

A more professional appearance is gained when using 35-mm slides, using single or dual projection facilities. Any of the presentation packages in the major software suites will produce output suitable for creating 35-mm slides. As the equipment for creating slides from a presentation package is expensive, it is usually found only in professional bureaux or in larger audiovisual departments. The files created can be sent by disk or via email to a bureau for creating slides. Each frame in the presentation can have a text note attached and the slide and note can be printed out on the same paper page as the speaker's notes. A number of slides can be printed out on each page to be used as audience handouts. The slides created for a presentation can be viewed on screen and the timings of the accompanying talk can be checked and refined. However, once created as 35-mm slides, it is expensive to correct errors or add extra slides. Although it is possible to extract slides from a variety of different presentations to create a new presentation with its own look, this new presentation would again have to be turned into 35-mm slides with the expense this would incur. The most widely used program for creating 35-mm slides is Microsoft PowerPoint, and as this is often the program that audiovisual departments use it is convenient to create the presentation in this format to avoid problems with file compatibility.

All the presentation packages will produce a screen show of slides with control over the timing and nature of transitions between individual slides. A means of demonstrating this directly to the audience produces a slick and professional presentation. Notebook computers have a port to allow connection to an external monitor and this can also be used to connect LCD panels which are placed over an overhead projector, and video projectors. Both are expensive and, as with any technology, prone to equipment failure. However, where available, this form of output allows use of both moving text and images on the individual slide together with sound output if connected to the auditorium sound system. As the use of PCs becomes ever more widespread and the equipment levels in auditoriums improve this will become the optimal means of giving a presentation.

With an eye to the developing potential of the internet, all the major programs produce output suitable for publication to web pages.

How to buy a PC

First considerations
- What will I want the computer to do in the future?
- How much can I afford to spend?
- Where should I buy?

What will I want the computer to do in the future?

This is a difficult question to answer today. Usually one's requirements increase in line with one's knowledge of the computer so try to buy a computer that is either in excess of today's requirements or that can be upgraded at a later date.

Remember that changes in the operating systems and software packages almost always place increased demands on the hardware. Windows Vista®, which was released in January 2007, requires a powerful graphics card and at least 1 GB of memory. It is said that you can never have too much of anything to do with the hardware side of computers. A browse through PC magazines or the internet will provide an up-to-date information on what the industry is currently selling as an entry-level model.

How much can I afford to spend?

As always, this is the limiting factor when buying a computer. In calculating your budget, remember to include the costs of any software and consumables (for example, disks, paper, ink cartridges). Many companies offer bundles of specific hardware and software that appear similar; look at the fine details and decide which package meets your needs closest. Some companies offer interest-free credit schemes from time to time, worthwhile as long as the bundle specified meets your requirements. On a limited budget, it is a good idea to spend the larger amount of money, in the first instance, on the parts of the system that cannot or are difficult to upgrade at a later date. The other parts can then be added or upgraded later. Remember the value of buying using a credit card for purchases over £100 in terms of the financial protection if the goods are not delivered.

Where should I buy?

There is now a wide range of retail outlets for computers, ranging from non-specialised high street shops to specialised computer dealers, as well as the internet . Mail order forms a large part of computer sales and it is also possible to hire computer systems.

Non-specialised high street shops may have good deals on specific systems but changing the specifications to suit your requirements may not be possible. It would be unreasonable to expect to receive the same expert advice there as you would in a specialised computer shop. The latter, besides offering better advice, tends to have a wider variety of computers available and should be able to tailor a machine to fit your requirements. A local shop is convenient not only to buy from, but also to return the goods for repair or upgrade. However, prices tend to be higher from a shop (in view of their overheads) than from mail order companies. Advice on a system to suit you may or may not be available from mail order companies but if you do know what you want they do offer cost savings and will usually configure a machine to your specific requirements.

All PCs will have at least a 1-year warranty on a return to base (RTB) basis, whereby it is your responsibility and cost to return the faulty machine to the vendor. Some companies provide an on-site service whereby a technician will come out to fix the PC, although there is a cost factor to consider – this may be 'built in' to the price of the PC. Independent support companies exist to provide this service, again at a cost. Some vendors offer 'extended warranties', for a price, for a number of years after the initial warranty period has expired. The value of these depends on the value of having your PC available and functioning at all times. For the average user, who has been clever enough to back up their data, a short time when the machine is returned to the vendor or even to a local shop for repair is an acceptable cheap(er) option. Bear in mind that there are very few parts that can go wrong – the most common being the hard disk, as it has moving parts, and the monitor.

Monitors
The standard monitor that comes with most PCs is now a flat-panel 17-inch or 19-inch TFT (thin-film transistor) LCD monitor. TFT monitors have almost completely displaced bulky CRT (cathode ray tube) monitors from the market as they take up so much less desk space and offer an extremely sharp and bright display. Their prices have fallen dramatically in recent years and even very large models (22-inch diagonal or more) are surprisingly affordable. Widescreen TFT monitors, which have a width-to-height pixel aspect ratio of 8:5 (e.g. 1680 by 1050 pixels) are increasingly popular. Another option, particularly for people who do desktop publishing and design work, who use very large spreadsheets or edit complex documents, or who do computer programming/application development, is a dual monitor system: many middle-of-the-range graphics cards now offer this.

Printers
The two main printer technologies are now inkjet and laser, both available with either black or colour printing. Dot matrix printers, which are cheap to operate but are noisy and produce lower quality output, have largely disappeared from the market. Inkjet printers offer almost laser-quality printout and are quiet. Printing times tend to be slow, especially for colour, although photo-quality output is now available and is relatively affordable. Lasers printers offer the highest quality printout but are more expensive to purchase.

Many printers are sold with a computer as part of a bundle, although these tend to be at the budget end of the printer range. Most of the leading manufacturers' products differ little in the quality or speed of printing when compared by price. However, to achieve the best quality output, specific papers and ink cartridges are required and the cost of these mounts at a surprising rate. For medium- or high-volume use, the cost of toner for a laser printer will be very much less than that of ink cartridges for an inkjet printer, and the higher purchase cost of a laser printer will be recouped within a few months.

Software
Software is an important part of the system, and is often not considered in advance. Decide what it is that you want the software to do for you, then which particular package meets those needs, then check that the hardware will run that package and, finally, find the money to buy it. Often, as with printers, a software package may be bundled with the computer. However, the benefits of a 'free £1000 worth of software' bundle may be less than expected if you never use any of this software.

Modems and the internet
To send and receive faxes or to access online information such as the internet, a fax-modem is required. These are either internal, which fit inside the machine and are cheaper, or external, which are more expensive but with indicator lights that indicate their connection status. Most new PCs are sold with an internal fax-modem; the standard speed is a 56 kbps (kilobits per second) modem. To access the Internet a contract with an ISP (internet service provider) is necessary. There are a variety of these providers and your telephone service supplier may provide this service.

Also available to the home user now are the much faster broadband connections provided by ADSL (asymmetric digital subscriber line). ADSL is a technology that uses standard telephone lines. An alteration is made at the telephone exchange and not all areas are currently serviced by an exchange that can handle the ADSL service. Also required is a splitter, which is plugged into the wall socket and separates the phone line into a normal line and the ADSL line, to connect to the ADSL modem. These modems are relatively cheap and connect via USB or, increasingly, ethernet, to the PC. As the line is split at the user's end, both the normal phone and the ADSL modem can be used simultaneously. ADSL connection speeds are now typically 4 or 8 Mbps (megabits per second).

A variety of connection packages are commercially available from the ISPs and many offer a combined telephone/mobile/broadband service, or even with cable or satellite television as part of the bundle. As well as the significant speed advantage, an ADSL connection is an always-on option and if heavy internet usage is expected then it would be the obvious choice.

Backup
The first three rules of computing should be: 1. Back up; 2. Back up; 3. Back up your data! Either the data created by the user(s) of the PC or the contents of the whole hard disk can be backed up. If the original program and operating system disks are available then backing up the data only will require significantly less storage space. It is also worth checking whether these disks are

provided when buying a new PC. It is significantly cheaper for the vendor to provide the operating system and programs preloaded without the original disks. In this case, the better vendors provide emergency rescue disks that will restore the PC to the purchased state when used. In this case, all the data created by the user(s) will be lost. There are a number of means of creating copies of data files, including copying to another PC, another hard disk (either internal or external to the PC) or to a removable disk such as a memory stick, DVD or CD-ROM. CD writer drives are now commonplace and DVD writer drives will store even more data. Whichever method is most appropriate, it is always a worthwhile form of insurance whose true value only becomes apparent when disaster strikes.

Finally

Remember that, as a result of the speed of change in the computer world, anything that you buy may well be obsolete within months. This need not be entirely depressing: as long as the system that you have bought suits your needs then it is the right computer for you.

Conclusion

This chapter has endeavoured to provide the non-computer user with an outline of the value of a modern PC with a suite of application software. The various software suites have not been described in detail, as the main functions are essentially identical with each other, with the differences being largely cosmetic. Detailed help on using the multitude of functions in each program is available on-screen, in the supplied manual or in commercially available guide books.

The particular software suite used is less important than actually having access to PC and software package to maximise the efforts of the individual researcher and enhance the end results of their efforts.

Glossary

ADSL Asymmetric Digital Subscriber Line. Uses the same copper wires that connect the telephone (for example at home) to the central telephone exchange of the local service provider. There is no interference with the telephone.

Application A specific task, such as stock control, for which a computerised solution exists.

ASCII American Standard Code for Information Interchange. A character encoding for relating a (binary) number to an alphanumeric character. The number is called the ASCII code. These are numbered 0 to 127, of which characters 32 to 126 are printable. Most operating systems and software now support Unicode, which offers a much wider range of special and international characters.

Background Refers to a non-interactive process running on a computer while the user is using another interactive process.

Backup Copying of files on to a storage medium for safekeeping in the event of damage to the original.

Backward compatible A program is backward compatible if it can use files from an older version of itself. For a file saved in the program to be backward compatible, it must be possible to open the file in a previous version of the program.

Boot To start up a computer system.

CD-ROM Compact disk – read-only memory. A CD-ROM is any compact disk that contains computer data. These disks can store up to 700 MB (megabytes). CD-ROM may also refer to the drive used to read these disks.

CD-R Compact Disk Recordable. A CD that can be written to using a drive that will write to compact disks.

CD-RW Compact Disk ReWritable. CD-RW refers to disks that can also be erased and reused to store data.

Character A single letter (A–Z), digit (0–9), special symbol (,.?< > ,etc.) or code used to control a device.

CHEST Combined Higher Education Software Team. Organises the bulk purchase and special deals of software for the academic sector.

Chip A piece of semiconductor material containing electronic circuitry.

Circuit A collection of electrical elements through which electricity flows.

Code The statements, either in compiled or text form, which make a program.

Command A user instruction to the computer, usually given via the keyboard but sometimes via a mouse or other pointing device. It can be a word or character that causes the computer to perform a specific action.

Compatibility The ability of a program, device or component to be used on more than one type of computer.

Computer network A set of interconnected computer systems, terminals and communications equipment.

Configuration The equipment making up a particular computer system or the initialisation commands given to a system before running an application.

CPU Central processing unit. Electronic components in a computer that control the transfer of data and perform logical and arithmetical operations.

Crash A catastrophic failure of a computer program, often owing to faulty logic in the program.

Cursor A movable, blinking bar of light on the screen marking the next point of character entry or change.

Cursor key Key used to move the cursor around the screen. Usually identified by an arrow on the key face.

Data Facts, numbers, letters and symbols stored in a computer.

Database A collection of organised data to be used for an application, for example personnel information.

Device A piece of hardware that performs some specific function. Input devices (for example keyboards) get data into the computer. Output devices (for example printers) get data out of the computer. Some devices are both input and output, for example memory sticks.

Disk A thin flat circular plate coated with magnetic material and used to store data.

Diskette A term sometimes used to refer to a floppy disk.

Display resolution Common screen resolution standards include the following:

    VGA: 640 by 480 pixels (now rare)
    SVGA: 800 by 600 pixels (now rare)
    XGA: 1024 by 768 pixels
    SXGA: 1280 by 1024 pixels

WSXGA: 1440 by 900 pixels (widescreen)

WSXGA+: 1680 by 1050 pixels (widescreen)

UXGA: 1600 by 1200 pixels

DOS Disk operating system. DOS was the standard operating system for PCs before Windows was created. It required the user to type commands at a boring screen with no pictures, no sound, no mouse and no colour. As time progressed, there were some good programs written for DOS that did offer these features (pictures, sounds, etc.) but each program usually worked in its own way, and you had to know DOS to get to the programs. Then Windows was invented. At first, Windows was just an add-on to DOS but now it is the standard operating system.

Dot matrix printer A printer that forms characters from a two-dimensional pattern of dots by pins striking an inked ribbon. Now largely obsolete.

Drive A device that holds a disk so that the computer can use the information stored on it.

DVD Digital Versatile Disk. Same physical size as a CD but can store 4.7 GB (gigabytes). This increased capacity is useful for storing video files, which require a lot of space. The recorded DVD can then be read either on a DVD player or a DVD-ROM drive on a computer.

Electronic mail (email) A way of sending memos or messages from one computer user to another.

Error message A textual message displayed when the computer encounters a problem.

File A file is a long sequence of bytes which represent data. Each file has a name and an extension which are separated by a dot (a period). The name, of course, identifies the file. The extension tells the computer what type of data is contained within the file. For example, a file called 'Letter to George.doc' is a Microsoft Word DOCUMENT.

File formats **.bmp** – a BitMaP graphics file native to Windows that does not support compression and thus files are very large

.eps – Encapsulated PostScript, a graphics file format

.gif – Graphics Interchange Format (pronounced jiff), a compressed graphics file format previously used widely on the internet but less so now as it only supports 256 colours

.jpg – JPEG (Joint Photographic Experts Group, pronounced jay-peg) is a commonly used standard method of compression for photographic images

.psd – Adobe Photoshop document

.tif – TIFF (Tagged Image File Format) is a widely used format for storing both photographic and line art

.wmf – Windows MetaFile, a graphics file format on Windows systems but no longer widely used

.doc – Microsoft Word document

.rtf – Rich Text Format, a file format developed for cross-platform document interchange: most word processors are able to read and write RTF documents

.ppt – Microsoft PowerPoint presentation

.xls – Microsoft Excel spreadsheet

.wma – Windows Media Audio, a compressed audio file format developed by Microsoft and intended to be a competitor to the popular MP3 format

.mp3 – a popular digital audio encoding format that includes effective data compression

.wav – a digital audio file format that

is usually uncompressed and can store sound in full CD quality

Filename The name assigned by the user to a file so that both the user and computer can read it.

Folder A folder can be thought of as a location on your hard disk or CD-ROM. Folders used to be called directories/subdirectories. A folder contains files and can contain nested folders (subfolders). Folders and subfolders are used to organise your hard disk. For example, you probably already have a folder named 'My Documents' on your hard disk; you could place a subfolder named 'Work' under 'My Documents' and place all your work documents within this subfolder. This way, you can keep your work documents separate from your personal documents.

Format (Verb) to format or initialise a disk to set it up ready to receive data. (Noun) a computer language statement which specifies the way in which output data are printed or displayed.

Function key Special key on a keyboard.

Graphics The use of lines and shapes to display data, as opposed to using printed characters alone.

Hard copy Output in a permanent form, usually on paper.

Hardware The tangible electronic (and mechanical) devices which constitute a computer system. This includes both the computer itself and any peripherals.

Icon An icon is a small picture used to represent an object. Some example objects are: data files, program files, folders, email messages and drives. Each type of object has a different icon. That means that different types of files each have an icon representing its file type. Microsoft Word files will have the Microsoft Word icon; Microsoft Excel files will have the Microsoft Excel icon, etc.

Inkjet printer A type of printer, which prints by controlling a jet or set of jets of ink so that the required shapes are marked onto paper.

Input Data entered into a computer.

Internet International network of networks.

JANET Joint Academic NETwork. A computer network interconnecting mainly academic users in the UK and with links to other computer networks abroad.

Keyboard The set of keys which allows characters to be sent to the computer when pressed. It inputs text and commands to the computer.

Laser printer A printer that uses a laser (or sometimes light emitting diodes or LEDs) to form its characters. Works very much like a photocopier.

Magnetic tape A thin tape coated with magnetic material and stored on reels. Only sequential access to the data is possible. This is a cost-effective form of backup for large organisations but is of little relevance to home users.

Mailbase A UK-based organisation which hosts mailing lists for the UK academic community.

Mainframe A physically large computer capable of manipulating large quantities of data and of supporting a number of concurrent users.

Memory The main high-speed storage area in a computer where a program is kept while it is being run. *See also* **RAM** and **ROM**.

Menu A list of options from which the user selects an action to be performed by entering a letter or moving the cursor.

Microcomputer A physically small computer, usually the cheapest type of computer.

Microprocessor A single-chip CPU.

Minicomputer A computer whose physical size lies between that of a microcomputer and a mainframe. It usually has a better performance than a microcomputer.

Modem Modulator/demodulator. A device that converts computer signals (binary data) into communications signals that can be sent over telephone wires.

Monitor A television-like device used for displaying data.

Mouse A peripheral device that is moved around a flat surface. The movement is translated into movement of a cursor around the monitor screen.

Multitasking The ability of a computer to appear to perform more than one task at a time, usually by giving small amounts of processing time to each task in turn.

Operating system A collection of programs which controls the overall operation of the computer. It performs tasks such as validating users, scheduling jobs, and controlling the peripherals.

Output Response from a computer, e.g. visual output on a screen, printed output, files written to disk.

Package A program or group of programs developed to perform a particular task, for example, statistical analysis.

Parallel interface A computer interface mainly used for connecting printers. However, many printers now connect via the newer USB interface.

PC (personal computer) A general term for a microcomputer designed for use by a single user at a time.

Peripheral A device that is external to the CPU and main memory but connected to it electrically, e.g. a printer or modem.

Printer A device for producing paper copies of data. *See also* **Dot matrix, Inkjet, Laser printers.**

Printout Refers to anything printed out by a peripheral or any computer-generated hard copy.

Program A collection of instructions needed to solve a particular problem or to guide the computer in its operation.

Programming languages The words and symbols, together with rules for combining them, that are used to construct computer programs. Usually these languages need to be translated into machine code before the computer can understand them. Examples are: COBOL, FORTRAN, BASIC, Pascal and C++. Languages can be high level or low level. The higher the level, the closer the language looks to English; the lower the level the closer the language looks to a list of mnemonics and numbers.

RAM Random Access Memory. Memory that can both be written to and read from. Its contents vanish when the computer is switched off. It is usually used to store the operating system, programs and their data while running.

Record A collection of related data items, e.g. the personnel record of an individual.

ROM Read-Only Memory. Memory that can only be read from. Its contents are permanent.

Screen The display surface of a monitor.

Serial A method of data transmission or an interface in which individual bits are sent one after another via a single signal or connecting wire. Serial interfaces are inherently slower than parallel ones.

Software Computer programs and data.

SPSS Statistical Package for Social Sciences – a statistical package widely used by users from all disciplines.

Stand-alone system A computer system that does not rely on other systems to perform tasks but may be linked by a computer network to any other computer.

System The combination of hardware and software making up a computer.

System disk A hard disk which contains essential information for booting a computer.

USB Universal Serial Bus. A standard bus type for all kinds of devices, including mice, scanners, digital cameras, printers and others. Devices can be connected and disconnected while the computer is on.

Tape streamer An input–output device for transferring data held on magnetic tape to and from a computer.

User The person who is using or operating a computer system or terminal.

User interface The set of prompts, commands, messages, etc., provided to a user to enable him/her to use a computer program or package. A command-driven interface is one where the user controls the program by typing in a sequence of commands in response to prompts. A graphical interface is one where the user controls the program by pointing at graphics (such as menus and icons) on the screen.

Virus A rogue program which can transfer itself from one disk to another be spread via email or be hidden in web pages. The virus program can then be triggered into action by certain commonplace commands or actions performed by the user. Some virus programs may simply flash messages or pictures on the screen, but others may corrupt program and data files.

Window A rectangular area on the screen that contains the interface between the user and a particular program. Several windows can be open at the same time, enabling a user to run programs simultaneously. Thus, a user might have a document displayed in one window, while running an application in another. Windows are usually associated with a graphical user interface.

Word processing A system that processes text, performing functions such as paragraphing, justification, paging, and printing out.

Write enable To remove write protection.

Write protect To protect a file or disk from having data written to it or removed from it.

WYSIWYG 'What you see is what you get', pronounced 'wizzy-wig'. It means that what you see on your screen while you edit your file looks the same as what you get when you print the file. Some older word processors were not WYSIWYG and formatting (such as bold or underline) would show up on-screen as strange codes (but look fine when printed). Today, ordinary word processors are almost always WYSIWYG; however, some software for creating web pages is not yet WYSIWYG.

WWW World Wide Web.

4

Effective literature searching

Lucy Reid and Elaine Garrett

Introduction

Searching for information and how the search is carried out is dependent upon the type of question being asked and why it is being asked. You may be trying to identify research topics, in which case you could:

- consult the consensus views of RCOG Study Groups or RCOG Green-top Guidelines
- consult the research recommendations of Cochrane Systematic Reviews
- search Cochrane CENTRAL for trials that have already been carried out
- search the National Research Register for continuing trials.

Having chosen your research topic, you might be searching for background information, in which case you could:

- search Medline for articles on epidemiology
- search Medline for the state of play in your chosen subject area.

Finally, you might be seeking evidence relating to the care of one particular patient, in which case you could:

- search pre-appraised sources such as TRIP (Turning Research into Practice database).

Formulating your question

Whatever you are searching for, it would be more effective to begin with a structured or clinical question. A clinical question converts the need for information into a form that can be answered from the literature. They are often known by the mnemonic PICO (Table 4.1).

All these elements will not necessarily need to be applied to each information resource searched but it is useful to have the components in mind before the search is initiated. Most information resources work best if the specificity of the search is built up in stages. Depending on the subject matter, the condition of the patient or the intervention that is being considered may be searched for first. Once this first broad search has been conducted, the results may be further specified by combining the search with another element of the PICO question.

Formulating a PICO-type question will also be of assistance when selecting suitable results. For example, you may find a paper that describes the

Table 4.1	Elements of a focused clinical question		
	Term	**Action**	**Example**
P	Patient	Identify salient details about your patient or population group. These might include sex, age range, diagnosis or symptoms	30-year-old primigravida with preterm prelabour rupture of the membranes at 33 weeks
I	Intervention	Identify the proposed treatment, diagnostic test or public health initiative	Antibiotics
C	Comparison	Identify a comparison or control against which your intervention can be assessed. This might be the current standard treatment or the gold standard diagnostic test	No antibiotics
O	Outcome	Identify your desired outcome, for example a term pregnancy, a quicker recovery period after surgery or better compliance with medication.	Prolonging the pregnancy, reducing maternal and neonatal infection

effect of an intervention on the same patient group that you are investigating. However, if the outcomes are significantly different from those you are hoping to achieve, the paper may be irrelevant to your search.

An unfocused question could be, for example: 'I need some information about preterm prelabour rupture of the membranes'. Alternatively, a clinical question could be: 'In a 30-year-old primigravid with preterm prelabour rupture of the membranes at 33 weeks, will antibiotics prolong the pregnancy and reduce maternal and neonatal infection?'

Once you have an answerable question, it is also advisable to spend a few minutes considering synonyms and alternative terms and spellings for the components of the question. This will ensure that the relevant information is retrieved, regardless of the terminology that the author has employed. For example:

- preterm prelabour rupture of the membranes
- preterm prelabour rupture of the membranes
- PPROM
- preterm rupture of the membranes.

General resources

Effective literature searching cannot be discussed without mentioning the internet. Every resource mentioned in this chapter is available on the worldwide web, so a certain familiarity with the technology is essential. As many people are comfortable with the web, there is no need to dwell too long on the basics in this section. If you feel your skills need to be improved, you could try out the following tutorials:

- BBC Webwise Online Course: provides an excellent introduction to the workings of the web and teaches how to navigate around the web effectively: www.bbc.co.uk/webwise/course/
- Internet Medic: a free online tutorial, which will introduce you to some of the medical resources available on the internet: www.vts.intute.ac.uk/he/tutorial/medic.

The internet is certainly a useful resource for clinicians, although any useful information is buried in a morass of irrelevant material. Deriving the most from the internet relies upon knowing how to locate relevant sources quickly and effectively. This section describes some approaches to identifying useful websites, as well as techniques for appraising the websites, to ascertain the quality of the information.

General search engines

One way to locate information on the web is to use a search engine. Search engines operate by creating databases of text from many different web pages. When a search term is entered, pages in the database that match your request are displayed. General search engines can be an effective means of searching information on organisations and people. They may also be used for searching for background information, images, news and discussion groups.

Google
www.google.co.uk
www.google.com

Google™ is one of the largest and most powerful search engines available. At the time of writing, Google indexes over eight billion items. One of the advantages of Google is its ability to index document formats such as PDFs (portable document format files) and Word documents, as well as web pages . It also presents the results in ranked order, so the most relevant information should appear towards the top of the results page.

To search Google, the relevant term is typed into the search box in the middle of the screen. Try entering the term 'pprom' and click on the **Search** button (Figure 4.1). Towards the top of the screen, you will see a breakdown of the search you have performed, together with an indication of how many sites have been retrieved. The results are then presented as a list of links. Each record includes the title of the page (which links directly to the page in question), a short paragraph from the page providing the context of the search term and the URL (uniform resource locator or web address) of the page.

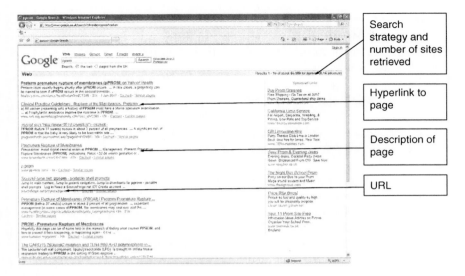

Search strategy and number of sites retrieved

Hyperlink to page

Description of page

URL

Figure 4.1 Google

There is also a link to a cached version of the page. This is the version of the page at the time it was last indexed by Google and can be valuable if the link has broken or the content has changed. Finally, there is an option to search for similar pages. Google will assess the content of the selected site and search for related pages.

As you scroll through the results of your 'pprom' search, you will notice that the information is derived from a wide range of sources, including hospitals, patient organisations and professional fora. You may have retrieved some references to journal articles and online textbooks. Google, and in particular Google Scholar, does index PubMed and the websites of individual publications. This can be useful but is not as effective as conducting a full literature search using standard bibliographic tools such as Medline. Finally, you will also notice that some of the items in your results are unrelated to your search, which is to be expected when using a general resource such as Google.

Carrying out simple searches using Google does produce some excellent results but, as with most database searching, these results are only as good as the search terms used. For example, in our earlier 'pprom' search, we will not have retrieved those sites that only use the full term: 'preterm prelabour rupture of the membranes'. To search for a phrase using Google, simply put your term in double quotes, for example "preterm prelabour rupture of the membranes".

Google supports the use of Boolean operators to combine searches, which is discussed in more detail in the Medline section below. The following exercise demonstrates how Google uses the Boolean operators.

Boolean searching

To search for pages which use either 'pprom' or 'preterm prelabour rupture of the membranes', enter the following in the search box (note that the OR must be in capitals):

pprom OR "preterm prelabour rupture of the membranes"

Google defaults to combining terms using AND; therefore, to search for 'antibiotic use and pprom', key in the following:

(pprom OR "preterm prelabour rupture of the membranes") antibiotic

Note that this will not retrieve items where the term 'antibiotics' is used nor will it find articles in which individual drug names are quoted. To include these, use the OR operator as above. The parentheses are also important as they instruct Google to carry out that section of the search before applying the 'AND antibiotic' element.

Occasionally, you will want to remove references to one term from a larger set. This is normally known as the NOT function but in Google the syntax is:

"rupture of the membranes – prelabour"

Try these and see what types of results are retrieved.

If all this seems slightly overwhelming, then access Google's **Advanced search** option. This provides a form that simplifies the process of creating complex searches and you can then use the drop-down menus to limit your search results by language, file format, date and so on.

Other searching

As well as the standard web searching facility, Google offers a range of other interesting options. The 'image search' facility allows pictures on the internet to be searched. Click on the **Image** link above the search box to access this facility.

While this function is useful, it is worth remembering that, as with most published material, websites are usually subject to copyright and images cannot be lifted and reproduced at will from other people's sites.

For other search options, including Google Scholar, click on the **more link** above the search box.

Finally, you may also like to refer to the **Advanced Search** tips for more information.

Although, Google has been discussed in this section, it is not the only search engine available. Other search engines may be preferable, so it is advisable to experiment with a range of them. Some alternative search engines are listed below:

- Yahoo: www.yahoo.com
- MSN Search: http://search.msn.com
- Ask: http://www.ask.com

Appraising sites

One of the problems of using general search engines is that you cannot be sure of the quality of the material that has been retrieved. Clinicians are accustomed to appraising literature and should regard information found on the internet with the same critical eye. It is worth considering that anyone can post items on the internet and that many sources are free from the high levels of editorial input that biomedical books and journals receive. Points of which to be aware include:

- The provenance of the information:
  - Is the author named?
  - Does the author provide his or her qualifications?
  - Is it clear who supports or funds the site?
  - Could there be any conflict of interest?
  - Is the information hosted by a reputable organisation?
    In some cases the URL of the page can give you a hint about this, for example as with the following suffixes:
    .ac.uk – academic sites
    .edu – academic sites
    .org – not-for-profit bodies
    .gov – government sites.
  - Has the information been subject to peer review?
- The currency of the information:
  - Is it clear when the information was written?
  - Has the information been updated?
- What type of information is it?
  - Does the site appear to give full, unbiased coverage of a topic?
  - How accurate is the information?

Medical search engines, gateways and portals

General search engines can retrieve large numbers of web pages but the quality of the results can vary. Consequently, search engines have been developed which only include material on defined topics, such as medicine. Whereas most general search engines use a high level of automation to gather data, specialist search engines rely more heavily upon subject experts who track down and index relevant pages. This increases the quality of the search results but the disadvantage is that the number of sites indexed tends to be relatively small.

Intute: Health and Life Sciences
www.intute.ac.ukhealthandlifesciences/

Intute: Health and Life Sciences (formerly the BIOME collection of gateways, which included OMNI) is a highly managed database of health-related web pages. Each entry is sourced, appraised for quality and indexed by information professionals. This means that searching the resource retrieves small number of hits but that the sites you find will mostly be relevant. As with Google, to search OMNI, the search term just needs to be keyed into the box in the centre of the screen (Figure 4.2).

Advanced searching is also available, which gives options such as searching by resource type (which allows the results to be restricted to patient information).

Subject headings may also be used to facilitate the search by using the **Browse** option. Subject headings, which will be discussed in more detail later in this chapter, enable you to carry out a single search which retrieves everything on a given subject, regardless of the terminology the author has used. A subject search for 'fetal membranes, premature rupture' will retrieve all relevant sites, including those referring to 'pprom', 'preterm prom' and 'preterm prelabour rupture of the membranes'.

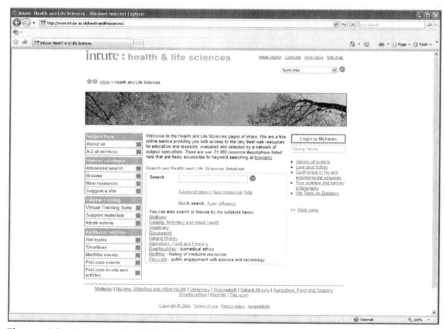

Figure 4.2   Intute: Health & Life Sciences

The National Library for Health and the Women's Health Specialist Library

www.library.nhs.uk

http://libraries.nelh.nhs.uk/womenshealth/

The National Library for Health is the NHS in England's gateway to high-quality healthcare information resources. It draws together a number of the resources that are mentioned here, and also provides access to other resources, such as the Clinical Evidence and the Core Content collection of databases and electronic journals. If you are a member of NHS staff in England, all these resources will be available to you. A password will be required to access some of them but the local healthcare librarian will be able to advise you further. Those working outside the NHS in England will still have access to some of the resources, so it is worth having a look at the site (Figure 4.3).

The other home countries of the UK also produce similar sites, which may be of interest:

- Northern Ireland: www.honni.qub.ac.uk
- Scotland: www.elib.scot.nhs.uk
- Wales: www.wales.nhs.uk

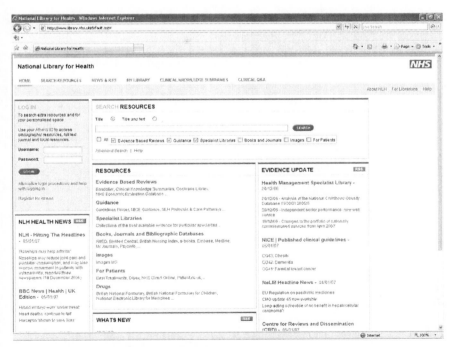

Figure 4.3   National Library for Health

Upon accessing the website for the National Library for Health, you will notice links to a number of specialist libraries. Each of these is designed to give easy access to high-quality evidence and information relevant to all professionals working in a specialty. The Women's Health Specialist Library indexes information on all aspects of obstetrics, gynaecology, midwifery and related topics. The site may be searched or browsed using the hierarchical subject menu on the left of the screen. Documents are sorted into resource type; for example, guidance and pathways, evidence and patient information (Figure 4.4).

TRIP
www.tripdatabase.com

TRIP (Turning Research into Practice) is a resource which allows you to search simultaneously across a range of other, high-quality, evidence-based internet resources in health care. These include query-answering services, guidelines, peer-reviewed journals and e-textbooks. To search TRIP, simply type your term into the search box. The operators AND and OR can be used to build complex searches. Some synonym searches are carried out automatically (Figure 4.5).

When you have carried out your search, results will be posted according to the type of information that they convey: evidence-based, guidelines, e-textbooks and so on. Click on the links to open results in a new window.

Geneva Foundation for Medical Education and Research (GFMER)
www.gfmer.ch/000_Homepage_En.htm

The Geneva Foundation is a not-for-profit organisation with links to Geneva University, the Geneva Medical Association and the World Health

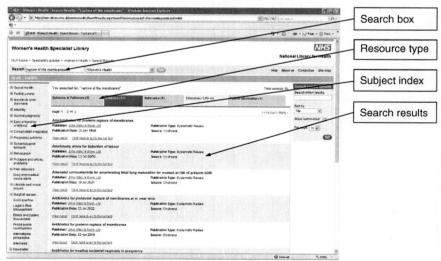

Figure 4.4 Woman's Health Specialist Library

Organization. It aims to promote education and research in reproductive health care, which is partly achieved by providing a gateway to relevant websites. The whole GFMER website provides interesting information but the most useful section is probably Databases and Links. This provides access to databases, full-text journals, guidelines and images (Figure 4.6).

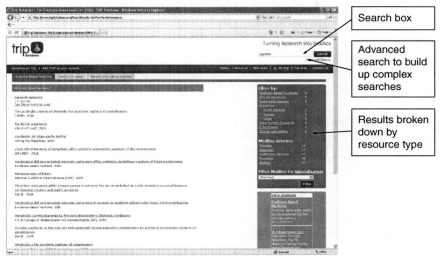

Search box

Advanced search to build up complex searches

Results broken down by resource type

Figure 4.5   TRIP database

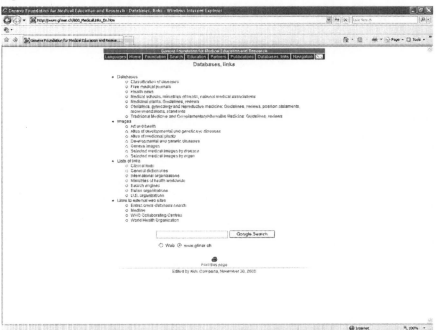

Figure 4.6   Geneva Foundation for Medical Education and Research and Research

Guidelines

Guidelines can be found through many of the sites already mentioned, such as OMNI and TRIP. They are also found on the websites of the organisations responsible for them, for example, the Royal College of Obstetricians and Gynaecologists (see www.rcog.org.uk). However, there are a number of resources devoted to indexing practice guidelines.

Specialist Library Guidelines Finder

http://libraries.nelh.nhs.uk/guidelinesFinder/
This resource indexes UK national guidelines and provides links to the full text where possible (Figure 4.7).

National Guideline Clearinghouse (NGC)

www.guideline.gov/
The NGC is the US central guideline resource. Most records take the form of structured abstracts of guidelines with either a link to the full text or a reference to the publication in which it appears (Figure 4.8).

Continuing clinical trials

It is often helpful to be able to find out what research is in progress but since most databases concentrate on published literature, this can be tricky. A couple of sites exist to help with this process.

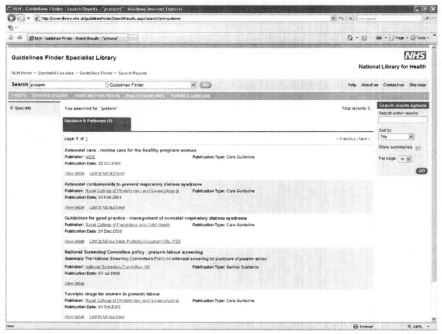

Figure 4.7   Guidelines Finder Specialist Library

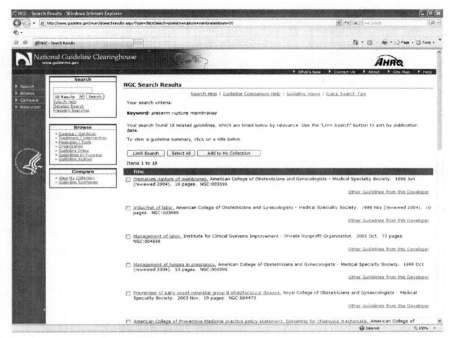

Figure 4.8 National Guidelines Clearinghouse

National Research Register (NRR)
www.nrr.nhs.uk/

The NRR is a database of continuing and recently completed research projects funded by the NHS (Figure 4.9).

ClinicalTrials.gov
www.clinicaltrials.gov/

This site is similar to the NRR, but indexes US-based research (Figure 4.10).

Statistics
You may wish to obtain background statistics before starting a research project but these can be extremely difficult to locate. A number of relevant sites do exist but locating the exact figures required can be time-consuming. The RCOG website includes links to various sources of statistical information (Figure 4.11).

Medline and bibliographic databases
Traditional bibliographic resources provide the most effective means of finding medical literature. The most well known of these is Medline but, depending on the subject of the search or the reason it is being conducted,

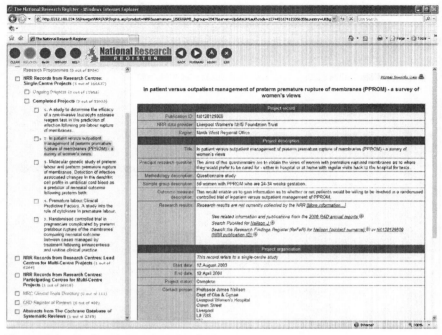

Figure 4.9   National Research Register

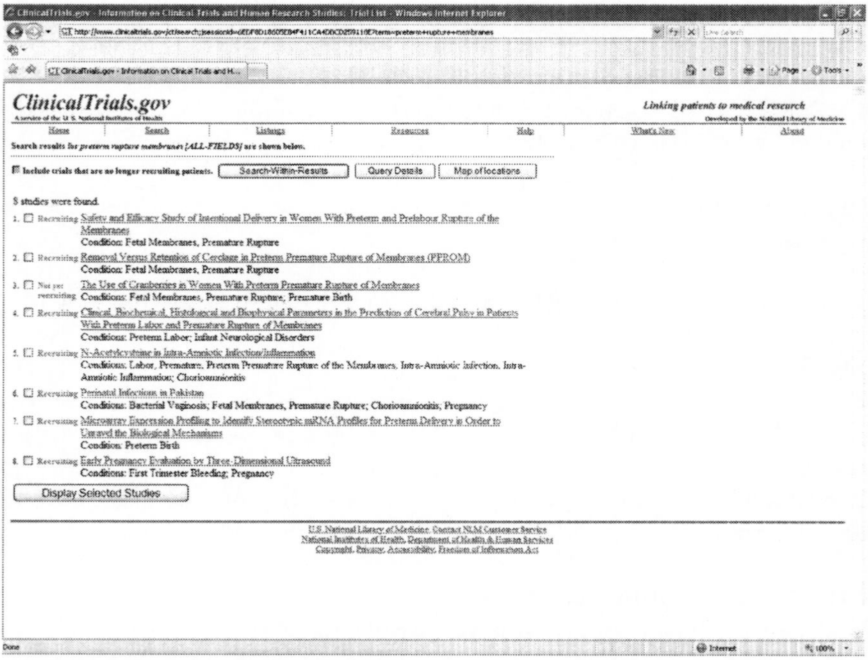

Figure 4.10   ClinicalTrials.gov

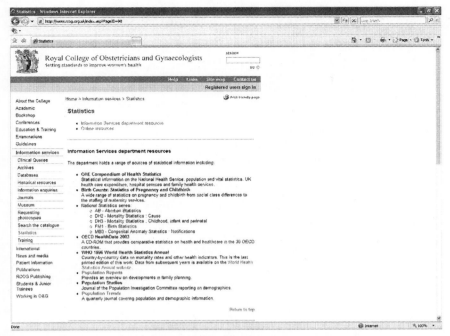

Figure 4.11 Statistics on the College website

other databases may be more relevant and may need to be considered. Table 4.2 lists some databases which may be used when conducting a search in this category, although there are many others. The general principles of searching most bibliographic databases are the same; this chapter will, therefore, concentrate on Medline.

Medline

There are several ways of accessing Medline. You may be familiar with PubMed (www.pubmed.gov), the free version, which is provided by the National Library of Medicine. Alternatively, you may use a service provided by Dialog or Ovid. Each of these interfaces is slightly different but the mechanics of carrying out a search will be the same. The Ovid interface will be used in this chapter. For assistance with using PubMed, refer to the following website: www.nlm.nih.gov/bsd/disted/pubmed.html. For assistance with using other interfaces, contact your local librarian.

You will be presented with a list of available data sets. To select one data set (for example, Medline 1966-present) simply click on the hyperlink. To select more than one data set, use the tick boxes to mark your selections and then click on **Continue**. Note that your searching will be more effective if you limit your selections to date ranges of the same database. Different

Database	Description	Period covered
Table 4.2	**Widely available biomedical databases**	
Medline	Produced by the National Library of Medicine in Washington DC. It covers about 4000 journal titles in all the medical specialties, plus some in nursing, veterinary science, psychology and pre-clinical sciences. Material from many countries and in many languages is included, although there is a slight North American bias	1966 to present time but material is being added to the Old Medline data set
EMBASE	Similar to Medline in that it indexes medical journals. However, it is produced by Elsevier and includes more European literature. It also focuses on pharmacological information but does not include any allied health material	1980 to present time
PsycINFO	Produced by the American Psychological Association and indexes books and journals in all psychology, social, behavioural and health sciences. It can be particularly helpful if you are looking for quality of life research	1806 to present time
CINAHL	Cumulative Index of Nursing and Allied Health Literature	1982 to present time
British Nursing Index	Like CINAHL, this indexes nursing literature but it has a UK bias	1985 to present time
HMIC	Produced by the Health Management Information Consortium and covers literature on the management of health care	1983 to present time

databases use different search terms and they are not compatible. Use the *i* buttons to access more information about the databases (Figure 4.12).

Subject searching

The example question considered earlier can now be subjected to Medline. The following example exercise indicates how the same question may be translated by Medline:

'In a 30-year-old primigravid with preterm prelabour rupture of the membranes at 33 weeks, will antibiotics prolong the pregnancy and reduce maternal and neonatal infection?'

As mentioned earlier, you should begin your search with one of the main concepts and build the complexity from there. Begin by entering the term

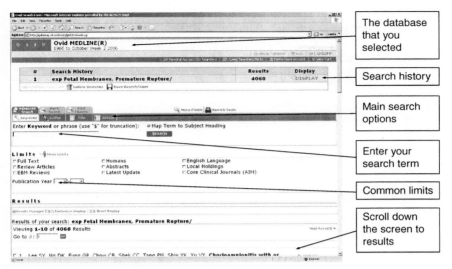

Figure 4.12 Ovid main search page

'pprom' into the search box, ensuring that the **Map Term to Subject Heading** box is ticked. With this box ticked, you are instructing the database to scan through its list of subject headings to present you with a list of options that match your concept most closely. Follow this by hitting the return button or click on **SEARCH** (Figure 4.13).

You will find that Medline suggests a number of terms (Medical Subject Headings or MeSH). You can use the tick boxes on the left to select the headings that are relevant. Be aware that, when selecting more than one heading, you will need to specify the way that the sets are combined. At the top of the screen there is a drop-down menu for the operators AND and OR. Using AND will give you the intersection of the sets. If you use OR you will retrieve all the results in the sets you have marked. For now, just select 'fetal membranes, premature rupture'.

To check the meaning of any of the terms, click on the *i* under **Scope**. This will provide a brief description of the coverage of the term, list synonyms and suggest alternative terms. When you are using a term for the first time, it is useful to check the scope to ensure it is the correct one. For example, the scope note for 'surgery' as a subject heading will inform you that it refers to the profession rather than the procedure.

Once you have selected your terms, you can opt to **Explode** and/or **Focus** your search. These instructions can be applied together as they are not mutually exclusive.

Focus
Subject headings may be divided into major and minor terms. An article may be tagged with 10–20 subject headings but two or three of these will be marked

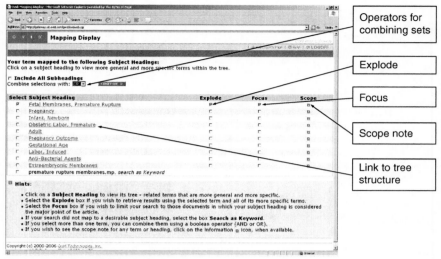

Figure 4.13   Ovid subject searching

as representing the main subject of the article. The **Focus** option allows you to search just the records in which your term is the major subject heading. This can be useful, especially in searches for common topics, but some relevant information could be lost, so ensure that caution is exercised when using this option.

Explode

Medical subject headings are arranged in a hierarchical tree structure. There are 15 top-level categories, such as anatomy, diseases, chemicals and drugs, each of which is further divided into successively narrower topics. Clicking on a hyperlinked subject term will take you to the tree structure and you can navigate around this hierarchy to find the term that most closely matches your search (Figure 4.14).

From the screen depicted in Figure 4.14, it can be seen that 'fetal membranes, premature rupture' falls into the category of 'labor complications', which also includes 'dystocia' and 'labor, premature' (note US spelling). It is also apparent that 'chorioamnionitis' is a narrower subset of 'fetal membranes, premature rupture'. The **Explode** option allows you to search for the subject term that you have selected and automatically include articles on any narrower terms that are available. In this case, exploding will include all references to 'fetal membranes, premature rupture' as well as 'chorioamnionitis'.

Once you have selected the relevant term of interest and opted to explode and focus as appropriate, click on **CONTINUE**. If you have chosen just one subject heading, the next screen will contain a list of subheadings. Subheadings can be used to qualify the subject heading that you have chosen. The *i* explains the scope of each term. If you are only interested in the epidemiology or mor-

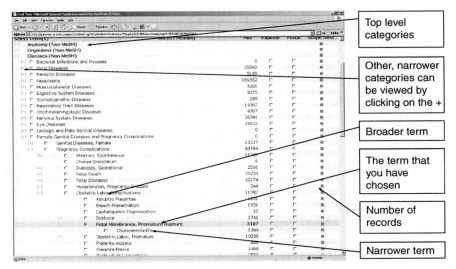

Figure 4.14 Ovid MeSH hierarchy

tality of PPROM then you can use subheadings to limit your search. However, if you are going to combine your search with other elements of your structured question then it is advisable to **Include all Subheadings** and continue.

You will now find yourself back at the main search page with the result of your first search appearing in the search history box. You may find it helpful to be able to decipher the syntax in this box, as it will enable you to work out the processes you have completed, so far. Also, note the number of records in each set to observe how the different searches affect the results (Figure 4.15).

Now carry out a second search for the second main element of our structured question: antibiotics. Remember to use the **Explode** and **Focus** options to include all types of antibiotics but to limit the results to articles in which antibiotics is the main subject.

Textword searching

Although medical subject headings are fairly comprehensive and initiating a search with them offers many advantages, on occasion, a more basic, textword search may still be required. A reason for this could be that the subject headings lag behind current medical thinking and newly discovered conditions and treatments may not yet have been assigned a subject heading. Another problem with the system is that the application of terms is subject to human error. If a literature search is being conducted for a systematic review, carrying out a comprehensive textword search should also be considered, to ensure that all the available information has been gathered.

To search effectively by textwords, you must first refer to the list of synonyms, spelling variations, acronyms and so on that was initially drawn up when you were formulating your structured question. With subject search-

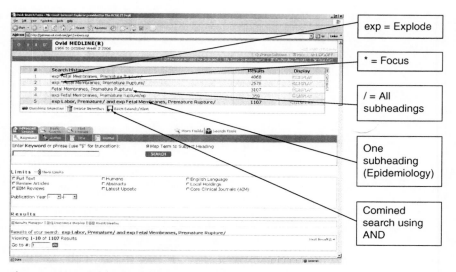

Figure 4.15 Ovid search history syntax

ing, everything associated with a given topic will be retrieved, regardless of the terminology the author has used. Textword searching does, however, rely simply on matching the string of characters that are searched for with those in the records. If you search for 'pprom' as a textword you will not retrieve articles where the author uses only the full term, "preterm prelabour rupture of the membranes", or "preterm PROM". (As we have already observed with Google, using speech marks around a phrase will force the database to search for the words adjacent to each other.) You will need to search for each of these synonyms and combine them into one big set by using the OR operator (see below).

Textword searching can be made more flexible by using wildcards. These replace various characters in words. In Ovid, for example, you could use the example in Table 4.3.

Another way of improving textword searching is to search for words close to each other. This gives a slightly broader search than the phrase searching (using double quotes) that we mentioned earlier but is still more accurate than searching for two words independently of each other. To carry out this kind of search, key the terms into the search box with 'adj' and the maximum number of intervening words . For example, 'prelabour adj4 preterm' will retrieve all instances of prelabour within five words of preterm.

You can perform a textword search in Ovid in a number of ways. The simplest method is to key the term into the usual subject search box, but before you click on **SEARCH**, make sure that the **Map Term to Subject Heading** box is not ticked. Another way is to key the term into the subject search box followed by: '.tw.' (e.g. pprom.tw.)

Table 4.3	Wildcards in Ovid	
Symbol	**Function**	**Example**
$	To replace a word ending	gynaecolog$ will retrieve gynaecologist, gynaecology and gynaecological
#	To replace one character	wom#n will retrieve women and woman
?	To replace one or no characters	labo?r will retrieve labour and labor
*	To replace a word ending	e.g. hysterectomy* will retrieve hysterectomy or hysterectomies
NEAR/	To find two terms within a given number of words of each other	e.g. preterm NEAR/4 rupture will retrieve instances when preterm and rupture occur within 4 words of each other

Author searching

On occasion, you may wish to check for papers written by a particular author. There are two ways of doing this:

- You can use the Author tab just above the search box. This will allow you to search an alphabetical list of all the authors indexed in Medline.
- Key the name into the search box followed by: .au. (e.g. Templeton AA.au.)

The format for author names is standardised to surname and initials but be aware that some authors do not use all their initials in every publication. If you are not sure what initials an author might have used you can key in: 'Templeton $.au.' to find anything by an author with that surname (see above for more information on wildcards.)

Journal title searching

You may also want to search for items in a particular journal. As with author searches, you can either use the **Journal** tab above the search box or key the title into the search box followed by: .jn. (e.g. lancet.jn.)

Remember that journals sometimes change their names. Medline usually indexes the full title of the journal so: 'bjog.jn.' will not retrieve any hits, whereas 'bjog $.jn' will find hundreds because the official title of the publication is *BJOG: An International Journal of Obstetrics and Gynaecology.*

Combining searches

You should now have two or more stand-alone searches. Your next task is to combine the two searches to retrieve papers in which 'pprom' and 'antibiotics' are both mentioned.

The most obvious way of conducting this search is to click on the **Combine Searches** button underneath the search history box. This will take you to a screen in which your search appears with tick boxes to the left of each line. Select the searches you want to combine, the operator you want to use and click on **Continue**. Another method is simply to type the instruction into the search box and then to press the return key or click on **SEARCH**: 1 and 2. There are three operators available in this method: AND, OR and NOT. The effect of these operators can be seen in Figure 4.16.

Limits

There are a number of limits that you may wish to apply to your search results. The most commonly used limits, such as **Review Articles** and **English language**, are available just below the main search box and can be applied before or after carrying out a search. Limits are applied to the highlighted search on your search history, usually the most recent one. Use the **Reset Display** button to retrieve and limit an earlier search.

Click on the **More Limits** button to apply other limits. The **Clinical Queries** option is one of the newest limits. Medline will filter your results for the forms of evidence that are most appropriate for the type of question being asked (therapy, diagnosis, etc.). Try applying the **Therapy (Optimized)** limit to our current search.

You will notice that most of the records retrieved refer to randomised controlled trials.

Viewing your results

Scroll down the page to see the first ten results from your set. The default position is set to view just the citation for each record.

To view the abstracts, you can either click on the **Abstract** link to the right of each record or use the **Customise Display** button to change the settings for the whole search session.

As you work your way through the results, you will find that some are more useful than others. You can mark those that you find particularly relevant by ticking the boxes on the left-hand side of the record.

Results Manager

When you have reached the end of your set, you can output the articles in which you are most interested by using the **Results Manager**. This allows you to print or save the results of your search or email them to yourself. Simply follow the instructions on the screen. It is advisable to keep a record of your search history so that you are aware of how the results were initially located.

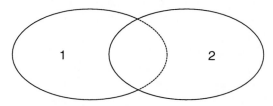

Figure 4.16 Boolean operators explained

Saving your search history

Finally, you may wish to save the steps of your search to use later. Click on the **Save Searche/Alert** button under the search history box. If you have not already done so, you will be prompted to set up a personal account, which provides a certain amount of disk space on which your histories will be saved.

Once you have set up a personal account, you will be able to save your searches temporarily (for 24 hours), permanently or as an **AutoAlert**. AutoAlerts are searches which are run automatically every time the database is updated (usually weekly). You will then receive an email informing you of any new records that match your search. If a search is to make a good AutoAlert it should have been carried out in a database which is going to be updated (i.e. the most recent one) and the search must be open ended (i.e. the last line must not resemble the following: "from 7 keep 1,3–4,15", as this can never generate new records).

The Cochrane Library
www.thecochranelibrary.com

The Cochrane Library is part bibliographic database and part full-text resource, housing, as it does, the full text of the systematic reviews published by The Cochrane Collaboration. For more information about the work of the Collaboration and the review process, access the following link: www.cochrane.org

The Cochrane Library is composed of eight different data sets, as shown in Table 4.4. As with Medline, the different components of the Cochrane Library are available through various interfaces. However, many people will access the Library through the publisher's website given above (Figure 4.17). This version is updated quarterly, although you may find that some of the databases are updated more frequently on other websites.

The basic principles of searching the Cochrane Library are the same as for any other database. You will need to build up your search by carrying out individual searches for each component of your focused question and then combine them to retrieve information relevant to your enquiry.

The most significant difference between the Cochrane Library and Medline is the application of subject headings. In common with many commercial bibliographic databases, Medline's strength is that every record added to the database conforms to certain stringent standards, which includes the use of a controlled vocabulary (MeSH) to describe the subject of the articles. As observed earlier, this allows for effective subject searching. Unfortunately, the application of subject headings is not standard in the Cochrane Library. This means that searching by MeSH, although useful for retrieving some records, is not effective across the entire database. To carry out a search of the Cochrane Library MeSH searching must be combined with textword searching.

Table 4.4	Components of the Cochrane Library
Data set	**Description**
Cochrane Database of Systematic Reviews (Cochrane Reviews)	Contains the full text of completed systematic reviews together with protocols of reviews which are in progress
Database of Abstracts of Reviews of Effects (DARE)	Produced by the Centre for Reviews and Dissemination at the University of York. It indexes systematic reviews produced by non-Cochrane bodies. Full records include a structured abstract with a commentary on the review. Provisional records include only the citation details
The Cochrane Central Register of Controlled Trials (CENTRAL)	Gives bibliographic details of controlled trials. It is the main register of trials that have been identified by the various Cochrane Review Groups. Many records have been collated from other bibliographic databases such as Medline but others have been identified by hand searching of reference lists and conference proceedings
Cochrane Database of Methodology Reviews (Methodology Reviews)	A very small database which provides the full text of systematic reviews of research methodologies
The Cochrane Methodology Register (Methodology Register)	Gives bibliographic references to publications about research methods which can be used in trials
Health Technology Assessment Database (HTA)	Gives details of continuing and completed reviews by members of the International Network of Agencies for Health Technology Assessment
NHS Economic Evaluation Database (NHS EED)	Indexes papers which include cost–benefit, cost–utility and cost effectiveness analyses
About The Cochrane Collaboration and the Cochrane Collaborative Review Groups	Gives information on the activities of the various Cochrane Review Groups

MeSH searching

To search using subject headings, click on the **MeSH Search** option towards the top right of the screen. A search box will appear into which you should type the subject that you are searching before clicking on **Go To MeSH Trees**. If an exact MeSH term has been entered, you will be presented with the relevant part of the hierarchical tree with your term highlighted in red. The number in the brackets indicates the number of narrower terms included in the one you have chosen. You can opt to explode your search to include any narrower terms. If you do not want to explode the search, select **Search this**

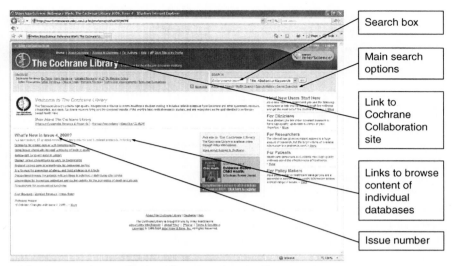

Figure 4.17 The Cochrane Library main search page

term only. To apply subheadings, use the drop-down menu entitled **Qualifiers**. To carry out the search itself, click on View Results.

If you are aware of the exact MeSH term, the database will try to map your search to available subject headings and will provide a list of sugges-tions. Click on the relevant suggestion to select it and then follow the steps described above to carry out the search.

Textword searching
As discussed earlier, textword searching can be more complicated then search-ing with subject headings. Every variation in terminology must be searched. There is also the need to be aware of spelling differences and the use of singu-lar and plural terms. Each of these will need to be searched and then com-bined using OR to create one large set comprising all the records on a given topic. You will then need to repeat the same process for the other elements of your focused question and finally combine each element using AND.

Fortunately, as with Medline, there are a number of actions that can be taken to make textword searching more effective.

Combining searches
To combine searches in the Cochrane Library, you will need to use the same operators that are used in Medline (AND, OR and NOT). These can be applied in an individual search string (for example, you can type 'preterm OR prelabour' into the search box).

To combine different lines of your search go to the **Search History** page where an outline of the searches conducted so far are listed. Key the search combination into the box (including the #) as follows:

#1 and #2

Then, click on **Go** (Figure 4.18).

Limits
A small number of limits can be applied to searches in the Cochrane Library. In both the **Advanced Search** and **Search History** screens you can limit your searches by publication date. You can also limit your search to new, updated or withdrawn records or those that have comments attached.

Viewing your results
Your search results will appear, broken down according to the individual data sets in which they appear (e.g. DARE, CENTRAL and NHS EED). To move between these data sets simply click on the hyperlink titles of the databases. The results are presented in pages of 25 and only the citation is available initially. To view the complete record, click on **Record**. You can mark your favourites using the tick boxes to the left of the screen.

Exporting your results
Individual records can be printed using the print option of your internet browser. To save your search results as a single file use the **Export** option. You can choose to save the citation alone or to include the abstract. You will then be asked to specify what kind of computer you are using. When you click on **Go**, you will be taken through the standard downloading procedure for your computer.

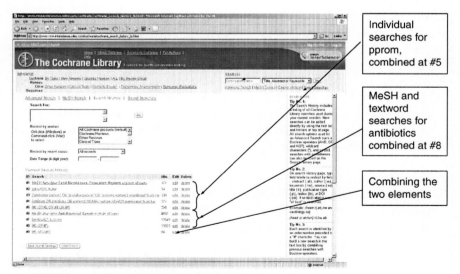

Figure 4.18   The Cochrane Library search history

Saving your search strategy

As with your Medline search, you may want to save the search process so that you can revisit it at a later date. Click on **Save Search Strategy** and complete the pop-up box with the title and description of your search. If you have not already done so, you will be asked to register with and log on to the Wiley site but this process is free of charge. Your search will be saved until you opt to delete it. The Wiley site does offer an automatic update service similar to Ovid's AutoAlerts but this is difficult to set up. A more effective way of retrieving new records matching your search is to rerun your search on a quarterly basis but also to ensure that it is limited to new records.

Cochrane Systematic Reviews

We cannot discuss the Cochrane Library without considering a Cochrane Systematic Review, as these documents form a major part of the database. Each review is structured in accordance with the strict guidelines stipulated by The Cochrane Collaboration. When a record in the database of systematic reviews is viewed it can be seen that the left-hand frame of the screen is taken up with a contents listing for the main document. The headings on this list are similar, irrespective of which review is being viewed. The contents listing can be used to jump straight to the part of the review that interests you most. There is also an option to download a PDF version of the review. You will notice that the body of the document appears in the main frame of the screen. This will start with the title, the authors and some information on how to cite the review. Next, you will find a structured abstract, which should provide a synopsis of the contents of the review broken down into standard headings.

Referring back to the left-hand menu, click on the **Figures** link to jump to that section of the review. In many reviews, each of the interventions and measured outcomes is shown on a graph known as a forrest plot, odds ratio diagram or blobogram. These diagrams provide an image of each of the individual studies which investigated the intervention along with a given outcome and the cumulated result of all the studies.

On first appearance, the blobograms can seem confusing but are relatively simple to interpret. The intervention and the measured outcome appear towards the top of the graph. The horizontal axis represents the probability that the intervention is effective. The vertical axis, which is known as the line of no effect, represents the point at which there is no difference between the intervention and the control. For each individual study you will see a square plotted on the horizontal axis. The size of the square represents the number of subjects involved in the study. The black line running through the square represents the 95% confidence interval: the range of results that you can be confident of achieving if you were to re-run the study across the whole population.

The findings of the individual studies are combined to produce a summary that includes all the results. Each of the smaller studies is weighted, usually based on the size of the study, and the results are amalgamated accordingly. By combining several smaller studies investigating the same outcome, the summary can provide a better representation of the population as a whole. The summary is represented at the bottom of the blobogram by a black lozenge. Again, the width of the lozenge shows the 95% confidence interval.

The results of the studies (whether there were more or fewer instances of a given outcome in the treatment or control group) are indicated by the position of the squares and lozenge. Studies, which recorded fewer of a measured outcome, are plotted to the left of the line of no-effect while studies which found more of the outcome fall to the right. Before interpreting the results you should remind yourself what the measured outcome is. If the aim of your intervention is to achieve an increase in term pregnancies, then you will be anticipating results that fall on the right. If, however you are measuring still-births, you will want the results to appear on the left. Fortunately, many blobograms now include 'favours intervention' and 'favours control', underneath the graph to assist in interpreting the results. If the results of the summary touch or cross the line of no effect, then it cannot be confirmed that the intervention you are investigating is effective (Figure 4.19).

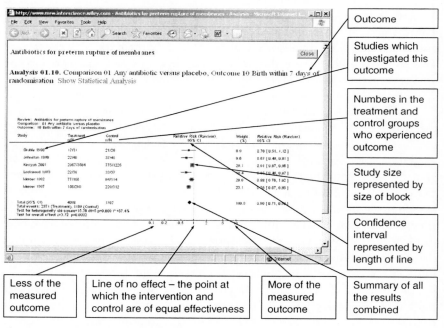

Figure 4.19 Interpreting a blobogram

Conclusion

We hope this chapter has provided enough information to give you the confidence to perform your own searches using a range of different resources. If you require help with any aspect of information retrieval, however, then do consult a librarian, who will be more than happy to help.

5

Critical appraisal of the research literature

Trish Greenhalgh

Research is the process of finding reliable answers to simple questions. Most biomedical research concerns quantitative studies (perhaps best exemplified by the randomised controlled trial) in which things are measured, counted and numerically compared with a view to confirming or refuting a specific hypothesis. In recent years, there has been increasing interest in the use of qualitative research, which adopts the techniques of the social sciences to gain an in-depth but non-numerical understanding of a particular topic and, perhaps, generate hypotheses that can then be tested in a quantitative study. Qualitative research is important but is beyond the scope of this brief chapter; its definition, application and limitations have been covered elsewhere.[1,2]

Critical appraisal is the process of looking at research findings with a view to answering three questions:

- Is this research valid (to what extent can I trust it)?
- Is it relevant (can I generalise the findings to my own practice)?
- What is the 'clinical bottom line' (should I change my practice and, if so, how)?

The research literature
Research evidence relevant to practising doctors usually falls into the category of either primary or secondary research evidence.

Primary
Primary (original and first-hand) research evidence comprises:

- randomised controlled trials: most commonly, those that compare the effect of a drug treatment with that of placebo or a competitor.
- cohort studies: in which subjects who have been exposed to a drug or toxin, such as a vaccine, tobacco or an environmental chemical, are followed up to see how many develop a particular disease or other outcome, compared with an unexposed cohort.
- case–control studies: in which subjects who have developed a disease, as well as control subjects who have not, are asked about their exposure in the past to a putative causative agent.
- case reports: in which a story about a particular event is told (most commonly these days, an adverse reaction to a drug).

- surveys: in which something is measured in a group of patients (for instance, their blood pressure) or a group of health professionals (such as their knowledge or attitudes).

Secondary

Secondary research evidence, which is of particular interest to the busy clinician, is material that sets out to summarise and draw conclusions from primary studies; for example:

- journalistic (non-systematic) reviews: which collect together some (but usually not all) primary evidence on a topic, usually interlaced with the author's personal opinion. Until recently, most overviews were written by experts in the field and presented in this format, which has been described as the tradition of 'eminence [sic] based health care'.
- systematic reviews: in which all the evidence pertaining to a particular field of research has been collected via a systematic search of the literature and unpublished sources and evaluated using predefined quality criteria.
- meta-analyses: which are systematic reviews in which the numerical results of different studies have been combined using standard statistical techniques; for example, the previously published meta-analysis of the association between obstetric complications and the subsequent development of schizophrenia.[3] Meta-analysis, simply by increasing the numbers in the calculations, can make the estimate of the effect of an intervention both more precise (the possible limits of its magnitude are more tightly defined) and more definitive (we can be much more confident that the result, whether positive or negative, is a true reflection of the effect studied rather than due to the play of chance).
- guidelines: which have been defined as systematically developed statements to assist practitioner decisions about appropriate health care for specific clinical circumstances.
- economic analyses: which are studies involving the use of mathematical techniques to define choices in resource allocation.

A piece of secondary research is only as good as the primary studies that went into it and the techniques used for making sense of those studies, so the notion that anything that bears the title 'systematic review' or 'meta-analysis' necessarily counts as high-quality evidence is erroneous. Similarly, most clinicians are all too aware that guidelines issued with the best intentions may or may not be valid or practicable. Current published guidelines for most conditions are based more on expert consensus than on primary research evidence.

Asking answerable questions

A preliminary step towards 'appraising the evidence' on a topic is to formulate a simple, answerable question before you start pulling articles out of the medical literature. The clinical epidemiologists have exhorted us to redraft

Table 5.1 The three-part question	
Question	**Example**
1. How would I describe a group of patients similar to this one?	'In primiparous women aged between 20 and 30 years and with no adverse family or personal medical history...'
2a. What intervention am I considering?	'... would planned home delivery ...'
2b. What comparison intervention am I considering?	'... compared with planned delivery by a midwife in a consultant-led obstetric unit...'
3. What are the most important and relevant outcomes?	'... lead to significant differences in maternal or fetal survival, neonatal morbidity, bonding and parental satisfaction with the birth?'

our clinical problems in the same language that researchers use to formulate their research hypotheses – that is, in terms of a three-part question,[4] as shown in Table 5.1.

Clinical reality, of course, rarely lends itself naturally to such clean and simple formulations. For example, a woman contemplating the options for the place of birth for her first baby probably incorporates around 100 different factors into her final decision, including:

- evidence about survival statistics and caesarean section rates
- values (her own and other people's), such as an overall attitude to 'natural' or conventional medicine
- anecdotal experiences related by other new mothers at antenatal classes
- even the presence or absence of an accessible car park at the hospital.

There is currently much debate in academic circles about whether it is useful to deconstruct personal health decisions into their component facts and values or whether we should accept that the paradigm of clinical epidemiology (the stuff of randomised controlled trials and their implications for individual patient decisions) can only address the simplest of issues and that the complexities of the lived experience of health and illness require a totally separate paradigm. Some authors (notably those whose specialty is decision science) argue that all health-related questions, no matter how complex, can be reduced to a series of dichotomous decisions, each of which can be addressed by a three-part question.[5]

Others, myself included, believe that the toolkit of clinical epidemiology, while invaluable for providing precise answers to oversimplified questions such as that in Table 5.1, ceases to be useful when applied to a complex real-life question such as 'where should **we** have **our** baby?'. The latter question should, in my view, be addressed by the couple themselves using an interpretative paradigm, by discussing the options and integrating their personal values and preferences with research-based evidence through dialogue and reflection.[6]

Whichever one of these theoretical standpoints you share, evidence has an important role to play. You will thus need to start with either a three-part question or some other structured and focused formulation and prioritisation of the clinical problems arising from the case. This is the step that is most often omitted in so-called evidence-based practice, resulting in what has been termed 'evidence-biased' medicine[7] (the foolish and naïve attempt to address one clinical question by means of research evidence that pertains to a different question).

Decide what sort of research evidence you need to address your question

Most clinical questions that arise from individual doctor–patient (or health professional–patient) encounters tend to be about interventions, particularly diagnostic tests (including the clinical examination itself as well as technical investigations) and treatments (including drug therapy, surgery, counselling and so on). Other important questions about individual patients include those about prognosis (what is likely to happen to a patient with condition X?). Questions arising from a public health or economic perspective may include practical issues of service delivery and the relative costs of different policies or protocols when applied to populations.

In general, questions about diagnostic tests should be answered by recourse to research studies that compare the test in question with a 'gold standard' in a defined, representative population. For example, the value of the quadruple test in prenatal screening for Down syndrome can be determined by offering the test to a sample of pregnant women and undertaking chromosomal analysis on the fetal tissue – either at amniocentesis or after birth.[8] The karyotype gives (or excludes) the diagnosis of Down syndrome with near 100% accuracy and the results of this test can be compared with those of the triple test to provide figures for:

- sensitivity (the extent to which the new test correctly picks up those with the condition)
- specificity (the extent to which it correctly excludes those without the condition)
- positive predictive value (if the test is positive, what the chance is that the patient actually has the condition).

These aspects of diagnostic test validation are discussed further elsewhere[4,9]

If the clinical question concerns a therapeutic (or preventative) intervention, the appropriate research design is virtually always a randomised controlled trial, or meta-analysis of randomised trials, for reasons that have been well rehearsed elsewhere[10] and are discussed later in this chapter.

Questions about prognosis are best answered not by randomised controlled trials but by a long-term (longitudinal) follow-up of a carefully assembled inception cohort. An appropriate cohort would be a group of individuals who share a particular feature (for example, a report of cervical intraepithelial neoplasia grade 1 (CIN1) on a routine cervical smear) who are then followed up to see what proportion recovers, stays the same or goes on to develop definitive disease. The prognosis of a condition as determined by a longitudinal cohort study will be heavily influenced by the sampling procedure. For example, a group of women in whom CIN1 is detected in sexually transmitted disease clinics may well have a different prognosis from women diagnosed with the same condition in general practice, mainly because of the presence of confounding variables (see below). Hence, you should pay particular attention to the first part of your three-part question, 'How would I describe a group of patients similar to this one?' when seeking prognostic evidence from cohort studies.

Many 'public health' type questions (that is, those that address the design and delivery of health care for a population rather than in an individual clinical decision) are also addressed through either randomised controlled trials or cohort studies. However, there is fierce debate about the ability of these methods to provide useful and practical answers to questions about community-based health promotion and/or models of service delivery. These complex issues, some authors argue, are better analysed using a qualitative or 'developmental' theoretical framework, in which lessons can be learned about the process of change as well as about final outcomes. These issues are not considered further here but the interested reader is invited to pursue the relevant references.[11-14]

Searching the literature

Having formulated your question, the next step is to make sure that you have the best evidence in front of you. A counsel of perfection would be to undertake a systematic literature search on your chosen topic, including the growing range of electronic medical databases, a hand search of the specialist journals, a search for recently published articles in the *Science Citation Index* and personal correspondence with leading researchers in the field[15] and with the pharmaceutical industry for negative unpublished papers. In practice, this process would take days or weeks and an acceptable compromise is to perform, with the help of a medical librarian if necessary, a search of the Medline, the Cochrane Library[10] and perhaps 'Clinical Evidence' databases,[16] using carefully selected subject headings and textwords. This step should take 2–15 minutes and will leave you with a manageable selection of articles to choose from.

Evaluating the methods section of published research: four pitfalls for the unwary

Table 5.2 shows a general checklist for evaluating the methods section of a research paper. A careful check through this list should detect the four main pitfalls in methodology: bias, confounding, power and validity.

Bias

Bias describes the systematic differences between groups that distort the comparisons between those groups. Bias is most obviously present in non-randomised trials in which comparison groups are allocated for convenience rather than at random – for example, all patients under consultant A receive one drug while those under consultant B receive a different drug. If consultant A's general approach to care differs from that of consultant B in important ways, differences in outcome would be wrongly attributed to differences in the efficacy of the drugs. Bias may also occur in randomised controlled trials

Table 5.2 Checklist for weighing up the methods section of a published paper (reproduced with permission from Greenhalgh, 2006)	
Question	**Check**
Was the study original?	
Whom is the study about?	How were subjects recruited? Who was included in and who was excluded from the study? Were the subjects studied in 'real life' circumstances?
Was the design of the study sensible?	What intervention or other manoeuvre was being considered? What outcome(s) were measured and how?
Was the study adequately controlled?	If a 'randomised trial', was randomisation truly random? If a cohort, case–control or other non-randomised comparative study, were the controls appropriate? Were the groups comparable in all important aspects except for the variable being studied? Was assessment of outcome (or, in a case–control study, allocation of cases) 'blind'?
Was the study large enough and continued for long enough and was follow-up complete enough to make the results credible?	

if randomisation is not truly random or if the allocation to groups is not concealed and if those assessing outcome are aware of which group the patient was in. The problems of bias in randomised trials are discussed further elsewhere.[10]

Confounding

Confounding is where a measured effect attributed to a particular variable is in fact due to an unmeasured co-variable. For example, as mentioned earlier in this chapter, patients recruited from a sexually transmitted diseases clinic may be more likely to have one or more current sexual partners than those recruited from a GP's smear clinic. Subsequent differences between the groups in outcome after treatment for CIN1 may be due to a difference in the interventions offered but may also be due to differences in sexual behaviour.

Power

Power is the ability of a study to detect a clinically significant difference between groups, if one exists. A trial should be big enough to have a high chance of detecting as statistically significant a worthwhile effect, if it exists, and thus to be reasonably sure that no benefit exists if it is not found in the trial. There is no need to memorise the formula for calculating the power of a study, which is described in most basic textbooks on statistics[17] and summarised in an online *BMJ* article.[18] It is important, however, to be aware of the three factors that influence the required sample size in a study: the nature of the primary outcome variable, the distribution of that variable in the study population and the size of a clinically significant change in that variable (what level of difference would you as a clinician deem important?).

For example, you might identify as a clinical problem the fact that a high proportion of infants born to Punjabi mothers who come to see you are underweight at birth and that many of these mothers are anaemic. In a randomised trial to measure the effect of iron supplementation, the outcome measure would clearly be the infants' birth weight but how many patients should you randomise? The answer will depend on how much variation there is in the birth weight of newborn Punjabi infants without any prophylactic intervention, a factor generally expressed as the standard deviation of the variable. You would also have to decide what is an important (clinically significant) improvement in weight. Would a 2200-g infant have a substantially better chance than one of 1900 g, 2100 g or 2150 g? There is no mathematical formula for determining what is clinically significant, which is why a statistically significant result may or may not be clinically relevant.

Validity

Validity describes the overall ability of the methods used to answer the research question. This aspect is often best addressed using a combination of specific clinical knowledge and common sense. Do the methods appear clinically sensible? Have the authors failed to take into account factors that you would have expected them to look at? Have they used appropriate equipment and drugs? If you were looking at this research question would you have done it this way? Whereas the aspects described above are often decided by a statistician or an expert in evidence-based health care, overall validity is generally best assessed by an experienced clinician who is familiar with the particular problem being studied.

Evaluating the results: defining the strength of evidence

The defining characteristic of 'evidence-based' therapeutic decision making as compared with traditional clinical methods is the use of mathematical estimates of probability and risk established from the average effect of the intervention in large population samples. It is beyond the scope of this chapter to discuss detailed statistical techniques for estimating such probability and risk, but clinicians should note some basic principles.

Until fairly recently, it was acceptable to look for the 'P values' in the results tables and count anything with $P < 0.05$ (less than one chance in 20 that this result occurred by chance) as a 'real' result. These days, P values are treated with increasing scepticism, especially when the number of comparisons performed by the authors exceeds about a dozen (making it quite likely that the result did arise by chance). It is generally felt that the results of research studies should not simply be classed as 'significant' or 'non-significant' but in terms of the likely magnitude of the effect of the intervention (point estimate of effect size) and the precision of this estimate.

The confidence interval around the effect size is, in effect, an estimate of the spread of results that might be found if the same experiment was repeated many hundreds of times. If the sample size was large, the actual result is very likely to reflect the true effect size. Conversely, small samples are more likely to produce extreme results through the play of chance. Hence, the larger the study, the narrower the confidence interval. If the confidence interval overlaps zero effect, either there is no real difference between the groups or the study is under powered – that is, a larger study (or a meta-analysis) needs to be done. A clinically significant difference between the groups and a confidence interval that does not overlap zero effect suggests that the study is both positive (there is probably a real effect) and definitive (there is no need to repeat it).

Results of intervention trials are increasingly expressed in terms of numbers needed to treat (NNTs). The calculation of NNTs and other commonly used summary terms for the results of clinical trials is shown in Table 5.3 and discussed in more detail in specialist texts.[19]

Conclusion

Critical appraisal skills are frequently equated with an 'evidence-based' approach to care. However, evidence-based practice is much more than the

Table 5.3   Illustration of mathematical estimate of benefit expressed as number needed to treat (figures taken from a randomised controlled trial which compared the effect of aspirin plus heparin versus aspirin in women with recurrent miscarriage and phospholipid antibodies.[23] The equations are explained in more detail elsewhere[19])

| | Miscarriage or stillbirth | | Total |
	Yes	No	
Control group (aspirin alone)	a = 26	b = 19	a + b = 45
Experimental group (aspirin plus heparin)	c = 13	d = 32	c + d = 45

Control event rate (CER) = risk of outcome event (miscarriage or stillbirth) in control group
$$= a/(a + b)$$
$$= 26/45$$
$$= 58\%$$

Experimental event rate (EER) = risk of outcome event in experimental group
$$= c/(c + d)$$
$$= 13/45$$
$$= 29\%$$

Absolute risk reduction (ARR) = CER − EER
$$= 58 - 29$$
$$= 29\%$$

Relative risk reduction (RRR) = (CER − EER)/CER
$$= (58 - 29)/58$$
$$= 50\%$$

Number needed to treat (NNT) = 1/ARR
$$= 1/(CER - EER)$$
$$= 1/0.29$$
$$= 3.4$$

This shows that between three and four women need to receive heparin plus aspirin in order for one more live birth to occur, compared with the outcome on aspirin alone.

ability to pick holes in published research papers. It is, many would argue, a way of thinking – an approach to systematically defining and addressing your own information needs and using that information appropriately and consistently in patient care.

Many practitioners would argue that the really difficult part of evidence-based practice is to do with implementation, either at the level of the individual consultation: 'Did I remember to consider appropriate contraceptive advice for 15-year-old Ms Jones after her termination of pregnancy and, if so, what were the attitudinal, ethical and practical influences on the application of so-called best evidence?' or, at the level of departmental policy: 'Having looked up the evidence to make a decision about Ms Jones, what general policy should we adopt in this department for responding to a request by an underage teenage smoker "to go on the Pill"?'.

The detailed analysis of how to implement change in professional practice and how to influence policy making for clinical effectiveness is beyond the scope of this chapter but this important subject is covered elsewhere.[20–23]

References

1. Mays N, Pope C, editors. *Qualitative Research in Health Care*. London: BMJ Publishing Group; 1996.
2. Greenhalgh T. Papers that go beyond numbers. In: Greenhalgh T. *How to Read a Paper: The Basics of Evidence-based Medicine*. 3rd ed. London: BMJ Publishing Group; 2006. p. 166–78.
3. Geddes J, Lawrie SM. Obstetric complications and schizophrenia: a meta-analysis. *Br J Psychiatry* 1995;167:786–93.
4. Sackett DL, Haynes RB, Guyatt GH, Tugwell P. *Clinical Epidemiology: A Basic Science for Clinical Medicine*. 2nd ed. Boston: Little, Brown and Company; 1991.
5. Dowie J. 'Evidence-based', 'cost-effective' and 'preference-driven' medicine: decision analysis based medical decision making is the pre-requisite. *J Health Serv Res Policy* 1996;1:104–13.
6. Greenhalgh T, Hurwitz B. *Narrative Based Medicine: Dialogue and Discourse in Clinical Practice*. London: BMJ Publishing Group; 1998.
7. Grimley Evans J. Evidence-based and evidence-biased medicine. *Age Ageing* 1995;24:461–3.
8. Wald NJ, Huttly WJ, Hackshaw AK. Antenatal screening for Down's syndrome with the quadruple test. *Lancet* 2003;361:835–6.
9. Greenhalgh T. Papers that report diagnostic or screening tests. In: Greenhalgh T. *How to Read a Paper: The Basics of Evidence-based Medicine*. 3rd ed. London: BMJ Publishing Group; 2006. p. 105–19.
10. Bero LA, Rennie D. Influences on the quality of published drug studies. *Int J Technol Assess Health Care* 1996;12:209–37.
11. Speller V, Learmonth A, Harrison D. The search for evidence of effective health promotion. *BMJ* 1997;315:361–3.
12. Britton A, Thorogood M, Coombes Y, Lewando-Hundt G. Search for evidence of effective health promotion. Quantitative outcome evaluation with qualitative process evaluation is best. *BMJ* 1998;316:703.
13. Greenhalgh T. Meta-analysis is a blunt and potentially misleading instrument for analysing models of service delivery. *BMJ* 1998;317:395–6.
14. Black N. Evidence based policy: proceed with care. *BMJ* 2001;323:275–9.
15. Chalmers I, Altman DG. *Systematic Reviews*. London: BMJ Publishing Group; 1995.
16. Clinical Evidence database [www.clinicalevidence.com].
17. Altman D. *Practical Statistics for Medical Research*. London: Chapman and Hall; 1991. p. 456.
18. Campbell MJ, Julious SA, Altman DG. Estimating sample sizes for binary, ordered categorical, and continuous outcomes in two group comparisons. *BMJ* 1995;311:1145–8.

19. Sackett DL, Richardson WS, Rosenberg W, Haynes RB. *Evidence-based Medicine: How to Practice and Teach EBM*. London: Churchill Livingstone; 1997.
20. Appleby J, Walshe K, Ham C. *Acting on the Evidence: A Review of Clinical Effectiveness: Sources of Information, Dissemination and Implementation*. Birmingham: NAHAT; 1995.
21. Oxman A, Davis D, Haynes RB, Thomson MA. No magic bullets: a systematic review of 102 trials of interventions to help health professionals deliver services more effectively or efficiently. *CMAJ (Ottawa)* 1995;153:1423–43.
22. Dunning M, Abi-Aad G, Gilbert D, Gillam S, Livett H. *Turning Evidence into Everyday Practice: An Interim Report from the PACE Programme, November 1997*. London: King's Fund; 1998.
23. Rai R, Cohen H, Dave M, Regan L. Randomised controlled trial of aspirin and aspirin plus heparin in pregnant women with recurrent miscarriage with phospholipid antibodies (or antiphospholipid antibodies). *BMJ* 1997;314:253–7.

Further reading

Field MJ, Lohr KN. *Clinical Practice Guidelines: Direction of a New Agency*. Washington DC: Institute of Medicine; 1990.

6

Evidence-based medicine and getting research into practice

Cindy M Farquhar

The term 'evidence-based medicine' (EBM) means integrating individual clinical expertise with the best available external clinical evidence from systematic research.[1] It was first described in the 1980s and, since that time, it has become an accepted approach to the delivery of quality health care, becoming integrated into many undergraduate, postgraduate and continuing education activities.[2] Centres for evidence-based practice have been established in many institutions, including clinical and academic and policy groups. The interest in EBM has occurred across a diverse range of specialties and backgrounds, including medical, dentistry, nursing, educational and purchasing personnel. One spin-off of EBM has been the increased interest in getting the evidence into practice. The most obvious way that this has occurred has been the development and implementation of clinical practice guidelines. The growth in the publication of guidelines mirrors the growth of EBM and there have been many studies showing the improvement in the quality of health care from clinical guidelines that have been implemented.[3,4]

The move towards EBM has also attracted some criticisms, which have ranged from describing EBM as 'old hat' to concerns that it is merely serving health rationing.[1] Some fear that it may interfere with individual clinicians' decisions by imposing rigid protocols and there have been medico-legal concerns raised. There have been concerns that research funding will be directed to health services research and away from basic sciences.[5] Critics of EBM have also pointed out that it is one thing to produce evidence but it is an entirely different matter to show that it changes practice and then an even greater step to show that it changes patient outcomes. Yet there are increasing numbers of examples of research influencing practice, provided it is not left to simple dissemination within the pages of a paper journal. Incorporating research findings into systematic reviews that are accurate, accessible and continually updated, as is the case with the Cochrane Library, is a huge step forward. Other approaches such as Clinical Evidence, which produces helpful brief summaries based on systematic review or randomised controlled trials (RCTs), are also useful in getting evidence into everyday care.

Evidence-based medicine

Evidence-based medicine has been defined as 'the conscientious, explicit and judicious use of current best evidence in making decisions about the care of individual patients'.[1] It is about taking the best clinical evidence from systematic searching of the research evidence and translating it into individual expertise. To put it more simply, it is for those, medically trained or not, who want to put the results of scientific research into everyday health care (Box 6.1).

Box 6.1	Elements of evidence-based learning
Asking	Converting the clinical puzzle into an answerable question.
Accessing	Searching to find the answer to that question.
Appraising	Critically evaluating the evidence to decide if it is, and if so how, reliable and robust.
Applying	Extracting the useful information and addressing the thorny issues of generalisability to decide what clinical action is best.
Assessing	Evaluating the process to integrate this element into the quality improvement cycle.

(Adapted from Del Mar *et al.*[7])

The approach of simply publishing research findings is no longer considered useful, predominantly because of the overwhelming amount of literature, which tends to overshadow the important clinical studies on which practice can be based. For example, if you (a clinician) wished to find out the most effective medical treatment for heavy menstrual bleeding, you may read a review article written by an 'expert' recommending norethisterone. Within this article you notice a lack of RCT data. You remember one RCT on the use of nonsteroidal anti-inflammatory agents, which demonstrated effectiveness. However, basing management on one RCT may be misleading – the quality of the trial needs to be assessed (was the allocation of treatment concealed? how did they assess improvement?) and the type of patients included also needs to be considered: how did they define heavy menstrual bleeding? Therefore, you decide to go a step further and look at other RCTs of medical treatment of heavy menstrual bleeding. You search Medline and find over 40 RCTs on the topic. How do you cope with this volume of research? Should all the papers be requested? Once the papers arrive how will their results be sifted and compared? It is a challenging task for any individual clinician to undertake in a short time frame. An alternative approach is to seek reviews of the evidence that have been systematically prepared by a group of independent individuals and peer reviewed. Many such reviews of clinical therapeutics are now being published and in particular these are the main focus of the Cochrane Collaboration.

The essentials of evidence-based medicine have been defined by Sackett and Haynes[6]. They include:
- asking the right questions
- finding the best level of evidence available
- appraising the evidence for quality and relevance
- implementing the results of the appraisal
- evaluating the changes in practice.

Asking the question

Almost every time a clinician sees a patient, new information will be needed about some element of their care. Some of the questions are obvious (what is the diagnosis?) and some are easy to answer from reference books (what is the safe dose?). However, often the questions will not be self-evident and time needs to be spent formulating the right question in order to track down the answers:
- Does this patient have risk factors?
- What is the prognosis for this condition?
- Which treatment is most effective in this particular patient?
- Which dosage is the most effective?
- Will this treatment cause more harm than benefit?

These questions are the starting point for using research evidence in everyday practice.[1] The essential elements of a clinical question are:
- Define which patients the question is about.
- Define which intervention and, if necessary an alternative intervention.
- Define which outcomes are of interest.

For example: Your patient is a 40-year-old woman with heavy menstrual bleeding wanting advice about medical or surgical approaches.

Which patients?	Premenopausal women with regular menstrual bleeding.
Which intervention?	Medical therapy (progestogen, nonsteroidal anti-inflammatory drugs, antifibrinolytic agents).
An alternative intervention?	Endometrial ablation or hysterectomy.
Which outcomes are desirable?	Reduction in heavy menstrual bleeding by pictorial bleeding assessment charts or patient satisfaction.

Finding the evidence

Finding the evidence is the next step. There are many electronic databases available, although Medline, PubMed and Embase are the ones most commonly used. The development of efficient search strategies for such databases has become a science initself.[8] Other sources of evidence include the Cochrane Library, which publishes a database solely of RCTs and controlled trials (mostly of interventions). It is the result of collaborative hand-searching efforts and electronic searching from many review groups and centres of the Cochrane Collaboration. This may be a good place to start, especially if therapeutics is the question about which you are interested. Most medical librarians are able to help with electronic searching.

Appraising the evidence

To be able to rely on evidence for clinical decision making, it is necessary to understand and appraise the study design and study quality. The appropriate study design depends on the research question (Table 6.1). For example, the question as to which is the most accurate diagnostic test for determining submucous fibroids in women is best answered by a comparative study of consecutive women with abnormal menstrual bleeding. A 'gold standard test' is compared with the new 'experimental test'. In the case of submucous fibroids, hysteroscopy is the gold standard and transvaginal ultrasound is the new test. The test should be conducted by two different observers who are unaware of each other's results and the data collected in a prospective manner. In the area of prognostics, the best research design includes repeated observations of individuals with an early-stage condition over a reasonable timeframe (longitudinal cohort study). For example, in order to study the natural history of simple and complex endometrial hyperplasia, repeated endometrial samples should be taken over a minimum of a 2-year period.

Table 6.1 The research question and the optimal study design	
Research question	**Optimal study design**
Diagnostics (Is this new test valid and reliable?)	Cross-sectional survey of new test and gold standard test
Screening (Should we use this as a screening test?)	Cross-sectional survey at pre-symptomatic stage of patients at risk
Prognostics (What is the long-term outcome of this particular diagnosis?)	Longitudinal cohort study of patients who have been diagnosed with early stage of disease
Causative (What are the risk factors for this condition?)	Cohort or case–control study
Therapy (How effective or harmful is this therapy?)	Randomised controlled trial or systematic review

In the area of therapeutic interventions, RCTs are considered the most powerful research design available to determine effectiveness.[9] Studies in which treatment is not allocated by randomisation tend to report larger, often false positive, treatment effects compared with randomised trials.[10] Not all interventions and treatments require RCTs. Sometimes, when the effects of care are dramatic, such research is unnecessary. For example, management of a woman with a severe prolapse will usually require a surgical procedure. Similarly, a woman who is repeatedly severely anaemic in association with heavy menstrual bleeding will probably benefit from a hysterectomy and a woman with an ovarian mass that is at risk of torsion or other complications is recommended to undergo surgical removal of the mass. However, where there is doubt about the best approach, for example the benefit of hormone replacement therapy in women with hot flushes, then RCTs are necessary to determine the harms and benefits. When more than one RCT is available, then a systematic review should be sought. In some instances, the differences between healthcare interventions may be the cost or adverse-effect profiles and these also need to be systematically evaluated. For example, in the management of endometriosis there is little discernible difference between the various forms of medical suppression on the outcomes of painful symptoms. However, there are notable differences when adverse effect profiles are taken into consideration.

One of the best sources of systematic reviews is the Cochrane Library. This is produced by the Cochrane Collaboration, which is focused on identifying reliable evidence and preparing systematic reviews of therapeutic interventions using RCTs. Collaborative review groups have evolved within the Cochrane Collaboration that cover most areas of health care. There are currently 51 Cochrane Review Groups internationally and seven of them deal directly with the field of obstetrics and gynaecology and women's health:

- Cochrane Pregnancy and Childbirth Group
- Cochrane Menstrual Disorders and Subfertility Group
- Cochrane Incontinence Group
- Cochrane Gynaecological Cancer Group
- Cochrane Fertility Regulation Group
- Cochrane Neonatal Group
- Cochrane Breast Cancer Group.

More than 400 systematic reviews relevant to the specialty of obstetrics and gynaecology are currently available on the Cochrane Library and a similar number are at protocol stage. A systematic review is one in which a systematic approach has been applied to asking a research question, identifying all the relevant RCTs, extracting the data and creating a systematic report, which is usually published in scientific publications. Cochrane systematic reviews are available on CD-ROM and on the internet and are probably the best source of evidence currently available because the process attempts to reduce all possible forms of bias and to be kept up to date. There are also a number of secondary journals with structured abstracts and critical appraisals with summaries that also provide useful sources of information.

Applying the evidence

After assessing the quality of evidence, the clinician needs to consider the relevance of the evidence. In many cases, research has focused on outcomes that may be of interest to the researcher but are of no value in clinical decision making. There are many examples of this in obstetrics and gynaecology. For example, there are over 20 RCTs of women taking hormone replacement therapy (HRT) where the outcome of interest is lipid profiles, yet the real outcome of interest is morbidity or mortality from cardiovascular disease. An abnormal lipid profile does not necessarily equate with clinical disease. This point was highlighted by the improvement in lipid profiles in women on HRT but no impact was seen on cardiovascular disease.[11,12] Other examples are:

- the trials on the use of barriers as a prevention strategy for adhesion formation in subfertility surgery that fail to report pregnancy data
- the studies of menstrual blood loss reduction with medical management of heavy menstrual bleeding that frequently ignore patient satisfaction.

Another criticism of primary research is that studies often fail to provide evidence of adverse or rare effects of treatment. For example, outcomes such as venous thrombosis, heart disease, stroke, breast cancer and endometrial cancer were not reported in the early studies of HRT, yet these outcomes are important to the long-term health of women.

In many instances, there will be no reliable or relevant research evidence available to guide decisions about health care. Ideally, in these circumstances, properly controlled research should be undertaken and patients entered into these trials. As this is not always possible, the next level of evidence can be used in clinical decision making (Table 6.2).

Table 6.2 Hierarchy of evidence (source: National Institute for Health and Clinical Excellence, UK[14])	
Level	**Evidence**
1a	Systematic review and meta-analysis of randomised controlled trials
1b	At least one randomised controlled trial
2a	At least one well-designed controlled study without randomisation
2b	At least one other type of well-designed quasi-experimental study
3	Well-designed non-experimental descriptive studies, such as comparative studies, correlation studies or case studies
4	Expert committee reports or opinions and/or clinical experience of respected authorities

In therapeutics, this depends on large cohorts, which are often compared with a selected control group. It is important to note that the control group and the study group are likely to differ in their presenting symptoms or demographics in some aspect. One example of this bias is in the area of HRT, where the large cohort studies suggested that women would have a reduction in heart disease,[13] whereas, the Women's Health Initiative study suggested no overall benefit and some harm.[11] Finally, if no reliable case series or cohort

Table 6.3 Strength of evidence corresponding to each level of recommendation (source: National Institute for Health and Clinical Excellence[14])

Grade	Strength of evidence
A	Directly based on level 1 evidence
B	Directly based on level 2 evidence or extrapolated recommendation from level 1 evidence
C	Directly based on level 3 evidence or extrapolated recommendation
D	Directly based on level 4 evidence or extrapolated recommendation from either level 1, 2 or 3 evidence
Good practice point	The view of the Guideline Development Group
NICE Technology Appraisal	Recommendation taken from a NICE Technology Appraisal

Table 6.4 Categorisation of interventions in BMJ Clinical Evidence[15]

Category	Definition
Beneficial	Interventions for which effectiveness has been demonstrated by clear evidence from RCTs, and for which expectation of harm is small compared with the benefits
Likely to be beneficial	Interventions for which effectiveness is less well established than for those listed under 'beneficial'
Trade off between benefits and harm	Interventions for which clinicians and patients should weigh up the beneficial and harmful effects according to individual circumstances and priorities
Unknown effectiveness	Interventions for which there are currently insufficient data or data of inadequate quality
Unlikely to be beneficial	Interventions for which lack of effectiveness is less well established than for those listed under 'likely to be ineffective or harmful'
Likely to be ineffective or harmful	Interventions for which ineffectiveness or harmfulness has been demonstrated by clear evidence

studies are available then the decision is based on expert opinion or consensus opinion.

There are several different approaches to levels of evidence and grading recommendations. The National Institute for Health and Clinical Excellence of the NHS uses the system given in Tables 6.2 and 6.3.[14] *Clinical Evidence*, a publication of the BMJ, suggests a different approach, which also has merit as it directs the clinician to consider harms and benefits (Table 6.4).[15]

Assessing evaluation of impact

Ideally, the final step of EBM is to evaluate the impact of the new evidence on clinical care. To do this, data need to be available on aspects of delivery of care and on changes in patient outcomes. This evaluation should ideally be planned in advance, so that 'before and after' data can be compared. It is also important to look not only at these things in the short term but also to evaluate whether the initial interest and changes achieved are sustained over time.

Getting research findings into practice: guideline development

Gathering and publishing reliable evidence does not ensure that patients are always offered optimal care. Numerous discrepancies exist between what is considered to be the most effective care and what occurs in reality. Lack of knowledge of the evidence is not the only challenge and there are many barriers that prevent the right patient being given the right treatment in a timely fashion.

The development of clinical practice guidelines is one approach to getting research into practice; they are defined as 'systematically defined statements to assist practitioner and patient decisions about appropriate health care for specific clinical circumstances'[16]. They represent an attempt to assess a large body of medical knowledge into a convenient, readily useable format. Like systematic reviews, they gather, appraise and combine evidence. However, most go beyond a systematic review in attempting to address all the questions relevant to clinical decision making for a particular topic. Guidelines differ from decision analyses in relying more on reasoning and should offer a certain amount of flexibility. The real advantage of evidence-based clinical guidelines is that they should incorporate evidence from many different sources of research – diagnostics, prognostics and therapeutics.

Guidelines also have their detractors. There have been concerns that they restrict clinical practice and reduce it to a series of decision points; they provide only a middle level of practice instead of best practice; they are inflexible and unable to accommodate local conditions; and they are political acts by managers keen to introduce cost saving.

One of the most commonly asked question is 'Have evidenced-based medicine and guidelines resulted in improved patient care?' Fortunately, this question has been answered by a systematic review of RCTs and 'other robust designs' which demonstrated improvements in care and better patient out-comes.[17] All but four of 59 published evaluations of clinical guidelines reported significant improvements in care and patient outcomes. Determinants of suc-cessful guidelines were also assessed and the development strategy, the dis-semination strategy and the implementation strategy all influenced final patient outcomes. Guidelines that had been developed by those who were going to use them, that were linked to specific educational packages and that had patient-specific prompts at the time of consultation had a greater likeli-hood of succeeding.[17]

Clinical guidelines should also undergo critical appraisal in order to con-sider whether they should be used. In 1998, a research collaboration (known as the AGREE collaboration) commenced, which was focused on developing an appraisal instrument to assess clinical guidelines.[18] AGREE stands for 'Appraisal of Guidelines Research and Evaluation'. The AGREE instrument with 23 items for guideline appraisal is available at www.agreecollaboration. org.

Ideally, guidelines are developed by individuals who represent multidisci-plinary groups, who agree independently to review all the available evidence from research and produce a simple format for the use of practitioners and patients alike. The guidelines should be peer reviewed and tested and the evi-dence in each guideline should be accompanied by grading the levels of evi-dence. A useful clinical guideline should be based on scientific evidence from well-designed research that has been systematically assessed. The value of alternative practices should allow health practitioners, in a reasonably short amount of time, to make links between multiple options and outcomes. It is hoped that with consistent reporting of guidelines development that system-atic methods will prevail, making the guidelines literature more accessible and useful for guideline users.

Implementation of guidelines

Developing a guideline that is then ignored either by not being disseminated or not being implemented is a waste of resources. Guideline development should include a plan of the steps and options for dissemination and imple-mentation and a recommended time frame. Unplanned clinical guideline implementation that has not been tailored to the various audiences it is appli-cable to usually results in unsuccessful guideline adoption.

There are three levels of implementation change to consider:
- the practitioner–patient level; for example, changing clinician/patient behaviour and attitudes
- the systems level; for example, enabling clinicians to make changes easily by providing access to computer decision support systems
- the policy level; for example, by providing coverage decisions that enable access to health interventions.

What works in implementation of clinical practice guidelines?

There is no single answer to what is a successful implementation strategy, although the limited research carried out suggests that a range of approaches is more likely to succeed than a single approach. Ideally, the research literature should guide this phase of guideline development but methodological limitations of the research base mean that this is not necessarily possible. For example, problems of sample sizes, length of time required before data analysis can begin, resources issues and different health systems often mean that the research cannot be transferred or generalised to other settings. However, some interventions have been shown to be consistently effective while others have variable, little or no effectiveness. These are summarised in Table 6.5.[19]

Educational outreach visits

Outreach visits are also known as academic detailing. These are face-to-face visits by trained personnel to clinicians within their practices. This is the approach that the pharmaceutical industry has undertaken for many years and believes it to be worthwhile for influencing decisions about prescribing. Other groups have also used it such as in sudden infant death syndrome research to influence midwives about babies' sleeping positions.

Decision support systems and other reminders

Decision support systems include anything manual or automated that prompt health professionals to perform a clinical action. Examples are reminders about screening or laboratory reports where results to note are highlighted, follow-up appointment systems and stickers on charts. In particular, computerised decision support systems have led to improvements in doctors'

Table 6.5 What works and does not work in guideline implementation (adapted from Bero et al.)[19]

Consistently effective	Variably effective	Little or no effect	Unknown effectiveness
Educational outreach visits	Audit and feedback	Dissemination of educational materials alone	Financial incentives
Decision support systems and other reminders	Local opinion leaders	Didactic educational meetings	Administrative interventions
Interactive educational meetings	Local consensus processes		
Multifaceted interventions	Patient-mediated interventions		
Mass media interventions			

decision making on drug dosage, provision of preventive care and general clinical management of patients. The advantage of these systems is that they are fairly easy to implement and are available to clinicians at the time required (just-in-time reminders).

Interactive educational meetings

Interactive educational meetings involve the active participation of health professionals and workshops, small-group discussions, problem-based learning or a range of other approaches. They should not be passive learning environments.

Multifaceted interventions

Multifaceted approaches are more effective than single interventions. Combinations of audit and feedback, face-to-face educational outreach or visitation using opinion leaders, reminders, local consensus processes and marketing are more effective than a single approach as they will tap into different parts of the change process.

Mass media campaigns

Both planned and unplanned approaches can be successful in the mass media, although the effect on health services may be modest. The mass media is a potential means of reaching all audiences at the same time.

Audit and feedback

Audit and feedback is a process in which the clinical performance over time is measured (audited) and fed back to the clinician. It does not necessarily include recommendations for action and there may not be other comparative data. Audit and feedback are most successful if the clinician receiving the feedback recognises clinical practice must change, is able to change within a supportive environment and can respond to the feedback immediately.

Use of local opinion leaders

Local opinion leaders are people who are trusted by their colleagues to evaluate new medical information and technology and apply this to the local context. This context may be hospital or community based, regional or national. Local opinion leaders are approached frequently for clinical advice, they should have good listening skills and are perceived as clinically competent and caring. They should be able to influence clinical practice among their peers. However, RCTs in this area have not shown consistent results.

Local consensus process

The involvement of local healthcare providers in solving local problems and, in particular, analysing barriers that may not be otherwise apparent to those in central planning authorities is invaluable and can help tailor solutions, particularly if consumer input is included.

Consumer-mediated intervention

Consumer-mediated interventions can include anything that aims to change a clinician's behaviour by the intervention of the consumer. Providing consumers with written information about the findings of an evidence-based guideline can influence the questions they ask and the expectations they have about therapies and treatments.

Dissemination of educational material

Single dissemination of educational materials including recommendations for clinical care, audiovisual materials, electronic publications and journal articles appears to have only a small effect in altering practice if carried out in isolation. Dissemination of guidelines by postal mail-out alone is unlikely to be effective in influencing clinical behaviour, although it may raise awareness and knowledge of the guideline. Unfortunately, this knowledge does not necessarily translate into changes in clinical practice. It is, however, a necessary and useful adjunct within a multifaceted implementation process.

Didactic educational sessions

The standard educational approach of lectures, personal visits or workshops in which there is no explicit effort made to change practice has often failed to change performance. However, they are relatively cheap and easy to set up.

Incentives and penalties

Many incentives already exist within the health system that are designed to influence clinical behaviour; for example, additional fee charges for giving immunisation, removal of items for reimbursement and provision of funds for retraining, personal satisfaction, professional incentives such as accreditation or continuing professional development points, and receipt of personalised relevant data through the evaluation process. Clinician behaviour is less likely to change if there are disincentives to do so such as increasing workload, extra time required, no familiarisation, the need for extra resources and the need for specialised skills and equipment. Disincentives for consumers also exist such as complications and the need for travel.

Administrative interventions

Administrative or management interventions that encourage or compel health professionals to change their practices are used widely but are infrequently evaluated. These include removing barriers, such as requiring approval of a specialist for certain tests, simplifying order forms, as well as providing incentives.

What are the barriers to getting research into practice?

An assessment of the barriers to successful implementation should be considered at this stage. There are likely to be barriers at a number of levels and stages of the process. The barriers are also likely to be different according to different providers and situations. The following barriers to incorporating guidelines into everyday practice have been identified.[20,21] There may be:

- genuine disagreement about the quality of the evidence
- an inability to accept the concept of levels of evidence
- an over-riding concern about medico-legal issues (over-ordering and over-treatment)
- personal preferences
- economic constraints and financial uncertainties
- failure of guidelines to be easy to use
- failure of patients to accept changes in practice
- a lack of patient-specific feedback.

One author concluded that the successful introduction of guidelines needs 'careful attention to the principles of change management: in particular leadership, energy, avoidance of unnecessary uncertainty, good communication, and, above all, time'.[22] Although surveys of healthcare providers consistently report high satisfaction with clinical practice guidelines and believe that they will improve quality, there are concerns about practicality of guidelines and their role in increasing litigation and in reducing costs.[5]

References

1. Sackett DL, Rosenberg WMC, Muir Gray JA, Haynes RB, Scott W. Evidence based medicine: what it is and what it isn't. *BMJ* 1996;312:71–2.
2. Straus SE. Jones G. What has evidence based medicine done for us? *BMJ* 2004;329:987–8.
3. Grimshaw JM, Thomas RE, MacLennan G, Fraser C, Ramsay CR, Vale L, *et al*. Effectiveness and efficiency of guideline dissemination and implementation strategies. *Health Technol Assess* 2004;8:1–72.
4. Bethell C, Reuland CH, Halfon N, Schor EL. Measuring the quality of preventive and developmental services for young children: national estimates and patterns of clinicians' performance. *Pediatrics* 2004;113(6 Suppl):1973–83.
5. Farquhar CM, Kofa E, Slutsky J. Clinicians' attitudes toward practice guidelines: a review of fifteen years of surveys. *Med J Aust* 2002;177:502–6.
6. Sackett DL, Haynes B. On the need for evidence based medicine. *Evid Based Med* 1995;1:5–6.
7. Del Mar C, Glasziou P, Mayer D. Teaching evidence based medicine. *BMJ* 2004;329:989–90.
8. Dickersin K, Scherer R, Lefebvre C. Identifying relevant studies for systematic review. In: Chalmers I, Altman DG, editors. *Systematic Reviews*. London: BMJ Publishing Group; 1995.

9. Sackett DL, Haynes RB, Guyatt GH, Tugwell P. *Clinical Epidemiology: A Basic Science for Clinical Medicine*. 2nd ed. Boston: Little & Brown; 1991.
10. Sacks HS, Chalmers TC, Smith HJ. Randomisation versus historical assignment in controlled clinical trials. *Am Med J* 1993;309:1353–61.
11. Writing Group for the Women's Health Initiative. Risks and benefits of estrogen plus progestin in healthy postmenopausal women. Principal results from the Women's Health Initiative randomized controlled trial. *JAMA* 2002;288:321–33.
12. Espeland MA, Marcovina SM, Miller V, Wood PD, Wasilauskas C, Sherwin R, *et al*. Effect of postmenopausal hormone therapy on lipoprotein(a) concentration. PEPI Investigators. Postmenopausal Estrogen/Progestin Interventions. *Circulation* 1998;97:979–86.
13. Colditz GA, Willett WC, Stampfer MJ, Rosner B, Speizer FE, Hennekens CH. Menopause and the risk of coronary heart disease in women. *New Engl J Med* 1987;316:1105–10.
14. National Institute for Health and Clinical Excellence [www. nice. org.uk].
15. *BMJ Clinical Evidence*. BMJ Publishing [www. clinicalevidence.org/ceweb/conditions/index.asp].
16. Field MJ, Lohr ICN. *Clinical Practice Guidelines: Direction of a New Agency*. Washington DC: Institute of Medicine;1990.
17. Grimshaw JM, Russell IT. Effect of clinical guidelines on medical practice. A systematic review of rigorous evaluations. *Lancet* 1993;342:1317.
18. The AGREE Collaboration. Writing Group: Cluzeau FA, Burgers JS, Brouwers M, Grol R, Mäkelä M, Littlejohns P, *et al*. Development and validation of an international appraisal instrument for assessing the quality of clinical practice guidelines: the AGREE project. *Qual Saf Health Care* 2003;12:18–23.
19. Bero LA, Grilli R, Grimshaw JM, Harvey E, Oxman AD, Thompson MA. Closing the gap between research and practice: an overview of systematic reviews of interventions to promote the implementation of research findings. *BMJ* 1998;317:465–468.
20. Greenhalgh T. *How to Read a Paper. The Basics of Evidence Based Medicine*. 3rd ed. London: BMJ Publishing Group; 2006.
21. Carnett WG. Clinical practice guidelines: a tool to improve care. *Qual Manag Health Care* 1999;8:13–21.
22. Ayers P, Renvoize T, Robinson M. Clinical guidelines: key decisions for acute service providers. *Br J Healthcare Management* 1995;547–51.

7

Audit

Gillian C Penney

What audit is – and what it is not

The current 'official' definition of clinical audit is 'a quality improvement process that seeks to improve patient care and outcomes through systematic review of care against explicit criteria and the implementation of change. Aspects of the structure, processes and outcomes of care are selected and systematically evaluated. Where indicated, changes are implemented at an individual, team, or service level and further monitoring is used to confirm improvement in healthcare delivery'.

This definition is taken from *Principles for Best Practice in Clinical Audit*,[1] is endorsed by the National Institute for Health and Clinical Excellence (NICE) and has evolved from the definition first used in the *Working for Patients* White Paper.[2] This 1989 White Paper used the term 'medical' audit. During the intervening years, the broader term 'clinical' audit has been adopted. This change reflects an acknowledgment that audit should be a multidisciplinary activity. The definition conveys the recognised principles of audit: a systematic process addressing the three dimensions of care (structure, process and outcome) and based on a commitment to change.

Confusion over which evaluation exercises constitute 'clinical audit' and which constitute 'clinical research' remains common. Richard Smith, former editor of the *BMJ*, succinctly summarised the difference as 'research is concerned with discovering the right thing to do; audit with ensuring that the thing is done right'.[3] In other words, the purpose of research is to determine whether clinical interventions (whether for diagnosis or treatment) are effective and the purpose of audit is to determine, and to maximise, the extent to which effective interventions are successfully adopted into clinical practice.

Any exercise designed to determine whether a treatment is better than no treatment or whether one treatment is better than another is not audit – it is research. Any exercise designed to determine the extent to which a treatment of proven effectiveness is being used in a given clinical setting is audit.

Clinical audit, clinical effectiveness and clinical governance

Clinical effectiveness has been defined as 'the use of specific clinical interventions which, when deployed in the field for a particular patient or population, do what they are intended to do: maintain and improve health and secure the greatest possible health gain from the available resources'.[4]

This definition means that clinical effectiveness involves the use of interventions that combine efficacy (they have been shown to work in the context of research studies), appropriateness (they also work in the real world of patients and populations) and efficiency (or cost effectiveness).

Promoting clinical effectiveness (the use of interventions possessing the attributes outlined above and the rejection of interventions lacking these attributes) was the aim of a major quality initiative of the UK NHS Executive, launched in 1996.[4] Clinical audit was viewed as a fundamental component of this initiative. The principal role of audit within the clinical effectiveness initiative was to monitor current practice and to verify that change is occurring. However, well-conducted audit has a dual role: not only can it monitor change in practice but the process of audit itself, with feedback of results to participants, can also serve as a mechanism to promote change.

From 1998, clinical effectiveness became incorporated within a broader NHS quality initiative, clinical governance. The 'official' definition is as follows: 'A framework through which NHS organisations are accountable for continually improving the quality of their services and safeguarding high standards of care by creating an environment in which excellence in clinical care will flourish'.[5]

Clinical audit has stood the test of time and remains a fundamental component of this latest quality initiative. The publication in 2002 of *Principles for Best Practice in Clinical Audit*[1] jointly by the NICE , the Commission for Health Improvement (CHI) (now the Healthcare Commission), the Royal College of Nursing and the University of Leicester provided evidence for the continuing importance of clinical audit in the view of these national bodies.

Types and styles of clinical audit

Critical incident or adverse event audit

Confidential Enquiries into Maternal Deaths (CEMD) were introduced in the UK in 1952 and typify one style of audit. This approach, known as 'critical incident' or 'adverse event' audit, involves the identification of patients where an 'adverse event' (in this case, death) has occurred. The management of the identified cases is then reviewed, perhaps somewhat subjectively, by a panel of experts in order to identify substandard care and to learn lessons for the future. Reports on maternal deaths covering all the UK countries are published on a 3-yearly basis. At the time of writing, the most current report covered the years 2000 to 2002.[6]

This adverse event style of audit has subsequently been applied to other subject areas. The National Confidential Enquiry into Perioperative Deaths (NCEPOD) published its first report in 1989. This enquiry covers the UK (with the exception of Scotland) and aims to include all deaths in hospital within 30 days of a surgical procedure (excluding maternal deaths). The third report of the NCEPOD (published in September 1994) was of particular relevance to gynaecologists, as it included an appraisal of deaths following hysterectomy. This report was subsequently summarised for gynaecologists in a review article.[7] The review reflected on the aims of the NCEPOD, to examine clinical practice and identify remediable factors, and highlighted the incompleteness of the audit, with a rate of return of enquiry forms of 60% by surgeons and 61% by anaesthetists. Despite this incomplete coverage, the NCEPOD review of deaths following hysterectomy identified a number of recurring elements of substandard care. Low use of prophylaxis for deep vein thrombosis, poor attention to postoperative fluid balance and surgeons tackling operations with which they were unfamiliar emerged as particular areas of concern.

A final example of an adverse event audit is the Confidential Enquiry into Stillbirths and Deaths in Infancy (CESDI). The eighth annual report of CESDI was published in 2001.[8] Following the model of the other adverse event audits, CESDI aims to identify cases in which the adverse event of death has occurred. It covers fetal loss , stillbirths and deaths in the first year of life. Each year, CESDI selects a subset of these deaths (representing a group where remediable factors seem likely to be found) for detailed confidential enquiry. For example, in the fourth report, this subset comprised 'intrapartum-related deaths among mature, normally formed babies'.[9] Substandard care was identified in relation to 78% of these deaths. Over 70% of the instances of substandard care occurred during labour (with 19% relating to antepartum care and 11% to postpartum care) and over 75% of the instances related to the practice of obstetricians and hospital midwives (the main providers of intrapartum care). The main problem identified was the assessment of fetal condition by heart rate monitoring and blood sampling.

Since April 2003, the Confidential Enquiry into Maternal Deaths and the Confidential Enquiry into Stillbirths and Deaths in Infancy for England and Wales have been amalgamated within a new organisation, the Confidential Enquiry for Maternal and Child Health (CEMACH). CEMACH is funded by NICE and is continuing the work programmes of its two precursor organisations. In future, CEMACH will extend its remit to address deaths in children up to the age of 16 years.

Topic- or criterion-based audit

An alternative style of audit, described by Charles Shaw (then of the King's Fund) has been termed 'topic-' or 'criterion-based' audit.[10] This approach follows the steps of the now classic audit cycle (Figure 7.1).

The fundamental differences between the traditional, adverse-event style of audit and this more contemporary approach are as follows:
- In adverse event audit, quality of care is assessed, somewhat subjectively, by expert panels. In contrast, in criterion-based audit, care is assessed more

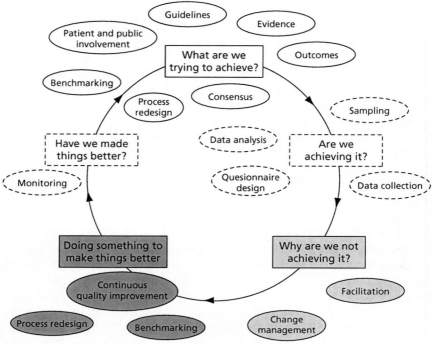

Figure 7.1 The audit cycle

objectively against previously agreed, explicit 'criteria for good-quality care'.

- The reviews of care undertaken in a criterion-based audit are objective and structured and they can be undertaken by non-expert audit assistants. This means that larger numbers of case records can be reviewed than would be possible within the expert panel approach of an adverse event audit.

Step-by-step guide to criterion-based audit

Criterion-based audit is, in general, the most suitable approach for small audit exercises at the level of the individual hospital or district. The remainder of this chapter is devoted to providing a step-by-step guide to criterion-based audit, with an illustrative example of a completed audit of this type.

Step 1. Pick a topic

As a general rule of thumb, the narrower an audit topic, the greater the likelihood of success. For example, an individual or small group of colleagues would be better conducting an audit of 'confirmation of ovulation among women presenting with infertility' rather than 'the management of infertility' or of 'provision of contraception following termination of pregnancy' rather than 'the management of termination of pregnancy'.

The choice of topic will be largely dictated by the interests of the instigating clinicians but a number of pointers should be borne in mind:

- The topic should be important in terms of its impact on patient wellbeing and/or its consumption of health service resources.
- Audit of the topic should be feasible. Feasibility is more likely if:
  - a sufficient research evidence base exists relating to the topic
  - there is a general consensus relating to the topic, presented in the literature and acceptable to the participants
  - the topic is amenable to the application of objective measurement
  - there is some indication that the topic is amenable to change if deficiencies are identified
  - sufficient resources are available (largely in terms of staff time and/or information systems) to conduct an audit of the scale and scope planned.

Step 2. Establish criteria for good-quality care

An audit criterion is a succinct statement summarising an element of good-quality care.[11] For example, in an audit of 'confirmation of ovulation among women presenting with infertility', an audit criterion might be 'a midluteal plasma progesterone level should be checked in a regularly menstruating female as the basic test of ovulation'. In an audit of 'provision of contraception following termination of pregnancy', a criterion might be 'if the oral contraceptive pill is chosen as the future method of contraception, pill-taking should begin on the day of termination'.

The examples above are of audit criteria relating to the process of care. Criteria may also relate to the outcome of care, for example '*in vitro* fertilisation should achieve a success rate of 15 live births/100 cycles commenced' or to the structure of services, for example 'gonadotrophins should only be prescribed in units which have access to ultrasound monitoring and estradiol assays 7 days a week'.

In general, it is most satisfactory to focus on process criteria. Process is usually easier to measure than outcome. If the process criteria used are evidence based, then good performance in terms of process should be reflected in good outcomes. For example, it is advised that contraceptive pill-taking should commence immediately following termination of pregnancy on the basis of research showing that a majority of women will resume ovulation within 28 days.[12] Thus, if a termination service achieves a high proportion of patients beginning the contraceptive pill immediately, this should be reflected in a good outcome in terms of a low proportion of women returning for repeat procedures. In general, audit criteria should be:

- objective and verifiable and therefore derived from scientific research (or consensus, if research evidence is lacking)
- capable of being measured
- acceptable to all participating clinicians.

Step 3. Agree on the standards to be met

Having agreed on a set of criteria against which the quality of care will be measured, clinicians may want to agree a related set of 'numerical standards' or 'target percentages' to be met. For example: 'among women who choose the oral contraceptive pill as their method of contraception following termination of pregnancy, 100% should begin pill-taking on the day of the procedure'. This step may be regarded as optional. Clinicians may prefer simply to measure practice in relation to the agreed criterion in a first round of audit and then to regard the performance achieved as the standard to be improved upon in a subsequent round. Thus, if it was found that only 75% of regularly menstruating women referred to a hospital clinic for investigation of infertility had their midluteal progesterone measured prior to referral, it might be agreed to accept 'better than 75%' as the numerical standard or target percentage for a subsequent audit period.

Step 4. Measure current practice

Having established criteria against which practice will be assessed (and, if desired, agreed target percentages to be met), the next step is to observe current practice. It may be possible to assess practice retrospectively using routinely collected information. For example, the Human Fertilisation and Embryology Authority (HFEA) routinely collects data on all IVF cycles undertaken. An individual clinic could, therefore, draw on this information to audit the outcome of care in its own service. More often, it is necessary to collect data, prospectively or retrospectively, specifically for the audit exercise. This may be done by a variety of means: by review of individual patient case records, by questionnaire survey of patients or by questionnaire survey of clinicians, asking them to describe aspects of their own practice.

For example, an assessment of the proportion of relevant women beginning pill-taking immediately after termination of pregnancy could be made by questionnaire survey of the women concerned. Conversely, assessment of the proportion of regularly menstruating women who had a midluteal plasma progesterone measured as part of the initial investigation of infertility might best be achieved by review of the patients' records.

As in a clinical research exercise, a formal sample size calculation should be performed to select an appropriate number of case notes for review or of patients or clinicians for survey. Appropriate selection of sample size will ensure that estimates of clinical performance are sufficiently precise. The freely available software package, Epi Info™, can be used to calculate sample sizes for single-group studies, such as audit exercises.

Step 5. Compare practice with the agreed criteria

Following measurement of current practice by the chosen means, the findings must be summarised to identify aspects of care which are satisfactory (by measuring up well to the agreed criteria) and for which changes are required.

For example, if all women who chose the contraceptive pill following termination of pregnancy were surveyed and all said that they had been provided with a supply of pills while in hospital and had taken their first pill prior to discharge, then it would be agreed that this aspect of care was satisfactory and no change was required. Conversely, if a review of the case records of women referred by their GPs for hospital investigation of infertility revealed that only 40% of those with regular menstrual cycles had had a midluteal progesterone checked prior to referral, it would probably be agreed that change was required.

Step 6. Implement change where indicated

Assuming that the audit reveals some aspects of care that measure up poorly against the agreed criteria, the next step is to promote appropriate change in practice. In choosing approaches that might persuade colleagues to change, it is important first to attempt to determine, for each deficient aspect of practice, the reasons for the deficiency. There are five principal explanations for care falling short of agreed standards:

- the agreed criterion is invalid or the standard set is unrealistic
- the organisation of care is deficient
- knowledge is inadequate
- skills are inadequate
- attitudes are inappropriate.

Sometimes the explanation for deficiencies may be glaringly obvious but, more often, teasing out the contribution of various causes may be difficult. However, since the purpose of audit is to bring about improvements this step must be tackled if the exercise is not to have been merely a waste of resources. The NHS Centre for Reviews and Dissemination has highlighted this type of 'diagnostic analysis' as fundamental in implementing evidence-based health care.[13] An analysis of the reasons for deficiencies in care and of the barriers to change leads to the design of interventions to promote change. Such measures might include:

- checklists (patient-specific reminders) to be completed by the clinician during, or shortly after, a clinical consultation
- the use of clinical guidelines, diagnostic algorithms, treatment protocols, etc.
- feedback to clinicians of audit results, indicating the extent to which current practice departs from the standards set.

Step 7. Repeat measurement of practice to confirm beneficial change

- Audit should not be merely a one-off observation of practice but should include repeat measurement, after an appropriate time interval, in order to monitor the extent of change. Knowledge of impending re-audit can, in itself, act as a stimulus to clinicians to introduce changes.

Ideally, an audit exercise should not comprise just the completion of an audit cycle as described above but should constitute what has been termed an 'audit spiral'. Measurement of practice is repeated on a number of occasions (with revision of criteria and standards if required owing to the availability of new evidence). It is to be hoped that such an audit spiral will demonstrate constantly improving standards of care.

Illustrative example of a criterion-based audit: three rounds of audit of the management of termination of pregnancy

A national audit of the management of termination of pregnancy was undertaken in Scotland. Two rounds of prospective, criterion-based, case-note review audit were undertaken in ten representative hospitals.[14] In addition, the outcome of care from the patients' viewpoint was assessed by questionnaire survey of women.[15] Following this national audit, one of the participating hospitals acknowledged that further improvements in termination of pregnancy care were required. After organisational changes within the gynaecology department, a third round of case-note review and a further questionnaire survey of patients was undertaken within this single hospital. The data collection methods and documentation were identical to those used in the national audit. The results of the successive rounds of this audit are presented here as an illustrative example of an exercise which progressed some way along the audit spiral.

Establishing criteria for good-quality care

A list of criteria for good-quality care relating to induced abortion was agreed by a combination of objective review of contemporary medical literature, panel discussions and postal survey of all consultant gynaecologists in Scotland.[16] The 11 criteria which were addressed in all three successive rounds of audit are listed in Table 7.1.

Measuring current practice

During each of the three audit periods, all women undergoing termination of pregnancy in the gynaecology unit were identified and data relating to the agreed criteria were collected by secretarial audit assistants by transfer of information from case notes on to a review document.[14] Each woman was asked by ward staff if she was willing to participate in a survey about her care. A questionnaire[15] was sent to the home address of each consenting woman four weeks following termination. It addressed the following topics: general satisfaction with care, provision of emotional support, provision of contraceptive advice and supplies, views on the availability of a choice of termination methods, follow-up arrangements and health problems following termination of pregnancy. Completed questionnaires were returned to the audit office using a stamped addressed envelope.

Table 7.1 Criteria for good-quality care agreed among consultant gynaecologists in Scotland and addressed in case-note review audit

Category	Audit criteria
Organisation of the service	1. All women requesting termination of pregnancy should be offered an appointment with a gynaecologist within 5 days of referral. 2 Termination of pregnancy should be undertaken within 7 days of the appointment with the gynaecologist. 3. In the absence of specific medical or social contraindications, women undergoing termination of pregnancy should be managed as day cases.
Pre-termination investigations	4. The woman's rhesus (Rh) status should be ascertained and Rh prophylaxis given following termination, if indicated. 5. Women undergoing termination of pregnancy should be screened for genital tract infection and treated if indicated.
Methods of termination	6. In selecting women undergoing surgical termination, a technique for cervical predilation should be used. 7. All surgical terminations at gestations over 10 weeks should be carried out by an experienced gynaecologist (post MRCOG or equivalent).
Post-termination care	8. Before being discharged, each patient should have agreed a contraceptive plan. 9. Before being discharged, each patient should be offered contraceptive supplies. 10. A follow-up appointment, either at hospital or with the referring doctor, should be given to every patient. 11. The follow-up appointment should be within 2 weeks of the termination procedure.

Data from the case-note reviews and from the patient questionnaires were entered into a computer database. Data from the successive rounds of audit were compared and statistical significance testing performed by chi-square analysis.

Comparing practice with the agreed criteria (and with practice during the previous audit periods)

During the 3-month local audit period, 389 consecutive patients were identified. Of these, 114 (29%) completed the patient questionnaire. Table 7.2 summarises the results of the case-note review relating to the 11 criteria. Results relating to

Table 7.2 Results in relation to 11 agreed audit criteria in three successive rounds of case-note review audit

Criterion	Element of care	National audit year 1 (n = 100)	National audit year 2 (n = 209)	Local audit (n = 389)
1	Percentage of cases seen within 5 days of referral	29	26	38a
2	Percentage of procedures undertaken within 7 days of clinic attendance	89	86	90
3	Percentage of patients managed as day cases	63	82a	82
4	Percentage of cases where Rh status recorded	99	95	100
5	Percentage of cases where genital tract bacteriology swabs taken	14	6	63a
6	Percentage of high-risk surgical abortions (> 10 weeks of gestation and/or age < 17 years) having cervical priming	69 (18/26)	86 (30/35)	92 (24/26)
7	Percentage of surgical abortions at > 10 weeks performed by senior registrar or above	55 (12/22)	75 (21/28)	92 (24/26)
8	Percentage of cases where contraceptive plan recorded	57	46	95a
9	Percentage of cases provided with contraceptive method by hospital staff	16	6	45a
10	Percentage of cases where follow-up plan recorded	25	52a	76a
11	Percentage of cases where follow-up within 2 weeks advised	4	35a	44a

a Significant improvement at $P < 0.05$ (chi-square test)

this series of 389 patients can be compared with those relating to the 100 and 209 patients studied in the same hospital during the two national audit periods.

Significant improvements (at the $P < 0.05$ level) had occurred since the second national audit period in relation to six of the 11 criteria. Patients seen within 5 days of referral rose from 26% to 38%; cases having genital tract bacteriology swabs taken prior to termination rose from 6% to 63%; patients for whom a future contraceptive plan was recorded rose from 46% to 95%; patients provided with contraceptive supplies by hospital staff rose from 6% to 45%; patients for whom a follow-up plan was recorded rose from 52% to

76% and those being offered follow-up within the recommended interval of 2 weeks rose from 35% to 44%.

Table 7.3 summarises the responses of the 114 women who returned outcome questionnaires for comparison with those of the 61 women (20% of those eligible) who responded during the national audit. Significant changes (at the $P < 0.05$ level) had occurred in relation to seven of 12 elements of care addressed. Patients indicating that they felt their decision had been right for them rose from 78% to 94%; those reporting that they received enough emotional support from hospital staff rose from 65% to 86%; those indicating that contraception had been discussed with them by hospital staff rose from

Criterion	Element of care	National audit (n = 61)	Local audit (n = 114)
	Table 7.3 Results in relation to patients' perceptions of care in two audit periods		
1	Percentage satisfied or very satisfied with care provided by doctors	88	84
2	Percentage satisfied or very satisfied with care provided by nursing and ancillary staff	92	93
3	Percentage indicating they had enough time and help in reaching their decision	78	90
4	Percentage indicating that (at 4 weeks post-termination) they felt their decision was right	78	94[a]
5	Percentage indicating that overall they received enough emotional support from hospital staff	65	86[a]
6	Percentage indicating that contraception was discussed with them by hospital staff	78	96[a]
7	Percentage indicating that contraceptive supplies had been offered to them by hospital staff	30	77[a]
8	Percentage who had adopted a contraceptive method at 4 weeks post-termination	88	88
9	Percentage indicating awareness of emergency contraception	66	88[a]
10	Percentage reporting that a follow-up appointment had been arranged	46	84[a]
11	Percentage indicating that they felt follow-up is worthwhile	78	93[a]
12	Percentage reporting post-termination health problems	27	20

[a] Significant improvement at $P < 0.05$ (chi-square test)

78% to 96%; those indicating that contraceptive supplies were offered to them prior to discharge rose from 30% to 77%; those who were aware of emergency contraception rose from 66% to 88%; those reporting that a follow-up appointment had been arranged for them rose from 46% to 84% and those indicating that they felt the follow-up appointment was worthwhile rose from 78% to 93%.

In the hospital described here, the results of a multicentre audit enabled clinicians to acknowledge deficiencies in their local service. In response to the audit findings, reorganisation within the gynaecology department resulted in the formation of dedicated pregnancy counselling clinics and in the appointment of nurses with responsibility for ensuring the smooth running of the termination of pregnancy service and for the provision of contraceptive advice and supplies.

Local staff undertook to monitor the effects of these organisational changes by means of a repeat audit resourced using local audit funds. It is encouraging that measurable changes in the quality of care, as assessed by both case-note review and patient survey, were demonstrable. Although response rates to the patient survey were, understandably, low on both occasions, it was felt that comparisons between the two time periods were valid.

This audit exercise, undertaken within a single hospital and using local resources, demonstrates the usefulness of clinical audit both in prompting changes in practice and in monitoring the impact of such changes. It is encouraging that a programme of audit initiated as part of a national exercise was continued at the local level, thus allowing progression along the audit spiral.

References

1. National Institute for Health and Clinical Excellence. *Principles for Best Practice in Clinical Audit*. Oxford: Radcliffe Medical Press Ltd; 2002.
2. Department of Health (DoH). *Working for Patients*. Medical Audit. London: HMSO, 1989.
3. Smith R. Audit and research. *BMJ* 1992;305:905–6.
4. NHS Executive. *Promoting Clinical Effectiveness: A Framework for Action in and through the NHS*. London: NHS Executive; 1996.
5. Scally G, Donaldson LJ. Clinical governance and the drive for quality improvement in the new NHS in England. *BMJ* 1998;317:61–5.
6. Lewis G, editor. *Why Mothers Die 2000–2002. The Sixth Report of Confidential Enquiries into Maternal Death in the United Kingdom*. London: RCOG Press; 2004.
7. Tindall VR. The National Confidential Enquiry into Perioperative Deaths. *Br J Obstet Gynaecol* 1994;101:468–70.
8. Confidential Enquiry into Stillbirths and Deaths in Infancy. *8th Annual Report*. London: Maternal and Child Health Research Consortium; 2001.
9. Confidential Enquiry into Stillbirths and Deaths in Infancy. *4th Annual Report*. London: Maternal and Child Health Research Consortium; 1997.

10. Shaw CD. Criterion based audit. In: Smith R, editor. *Audit in Action*. London: BMJ Publishing; 1992. p. 122–8.
11. Burnett AC, Winyard G. Clinical audit at the heart of clinical effectiveness. *J Qual Clin Pract* 1998;18:3–19.
12. Cameron IT, Baird DT. The return to ovulation following early abortion: a comparison between vacuum aspiration and prostaglandin. *Acta Endocrinol* 1988;118:161–7.
13. NHS Centre for Reviews and Dissemination. *Getting Evidence into Practice*. York: University of York; 1999.
14. Penney GC, Glasier A, Templeton A. A multi-centre, criterion-based audit of the management of induced abortion in Scotland. *BMJ* 1994;309:15–18.
15. Penney GC, Templeton A, Glasier A. Patient's views on abortion care in Scottish hospitals. *Health Bull* 1994;52:431–8.
16. Penney GC, Glasier A, Templeton A. Agreeing criteria for audit of the management of induced abortion: an approach by national consensus survey. *Qual Health Care* 1993;2:167–9.

8

Clinical trials

Siladitya Bhattacharya and Ashalatha Shetty

Introduction

The randomised clinical trial is widely accepted as a gold standard for the rigorous evaluation of treatments. Its principal strength lies in minimisation of bias, which allows clinically important effects due to interventions to be identified. This in turn helps to generate high-quality data, which can potentially lead to effective treatment strategies.

Terminology

The word 'clinical trial' is often used loosely to describe a variety of study designs. An 'uncontrolled trial' is essentially a case series of a treatment (usually new) without a control group. This type of evaluation is prone to serious bias, as practitioners often select patients in whom the outcome of a new technique is likely to be favourable. 'Controlled trials' represent studies where outcomes in patients subjected to the 'new' treatment are compared with those in a set of historical or concurrent controls in what is essentially a cohort design. Use of historical controls can bias the results in favour of a new treatment, partly owing to a more rigorous system of patient selection and partly owing to better systems of data collection for the new treatment.[1] Use of concurrent controls may also lead to erroneous results due to problems with self-selection of patients into experimental and control groups. The strength of clinical trials lies in true randomisation. Randomisation based on days of the week, odd or even unit numbers, are examples of 'quasi' rather than genuine randomisation. Tossing a coin, although theoretically sound, is unacceptable as there is considerable scope for bias and there is no audit trail.

Randomised clinical trials may be classified in a number of ways (Table 8.1). Some of these are discussed below.

Phase I clinical trials

Phase I trials are preliminary studies with an emphasis on drug safety, rather than efficacy, and may be performed on healthy volunteers. Most phase I trials are supported by the pharmaceutical industry and involve relatively small numbers of subjects. Protocols are strict and often involve extensive investigations for evidence of toxicity, including blood counts, biochemistry and liver and kidney function tests.

Table 8.1 Types of randomised clinical trials	
Trial type	**Randomisation**
Phased trials	Phase I
	Phase II
	Phase III
	Phase IV
Conduct	Pragmatic
	Explanatory
Design	Parallel group
	Crossover
	Factorial
	Patient preference
	Cluster
	Equivalence/non-inferiority
	Bayesian
Randomisation	True
	Quasi

Phase II clinical trials

Phase II trials are fairly small-scale investigations into the efficacy, safety, optimum dose and route of administration of a drug. All drug trials have to go through this phase. Examples include trials evaluating the use of misoprostol for medical termination of pregnancy[2] or initial trials of atosiban in tocolysis in preterm labour.[3]

Phase III clinical trials

Phase III trials evaluate effectiveness by comparing an intervention with the current standard management and/or placebo, in a large trial involving a substantial number of patients. Phase III trials represent the point of evaluation following which drugs and other interventions (including complex interventions) are introduced into clinical practice, such as the eclampsia trial and magnesium sulphate use.[4]

Phase IV clinical trials

Even after a new treatment finds general acceptance, unanswered questions about its safety and its long-term effectiveness continue to be asked. These are addressed in the context of Phase IV trials. For example, the long-term implications of new methods of treatment of menorrhagia, such as endometrial ablation, are still under evaluation a decade after the results of the first phase III trials were reported. Effects on the children 1.5 years after their mothers were administered aspirin in the CLASP trial[5] and maternal and infant outcomes 2 years after the Term Breech trial[6,7] are being evaluated.

Pragmatic and explanatory trials

Explanatory trials measure efficacy: the benefit produced by a treatment under ideal conditions. Pragmatic trials measure effectiveness: the benefit a treatment produces in routine clinical practice.[8] The aim of an explanatory trial is to assess the outcome of a new drug under controlled conditions using a homogeneous group of patients. Eligibility criteria are strict and protocol violations are not permitted. For example, in an explanatory trial evaluating an oral contraceptive pill or a tocolytic agent, women who fail to receive the appropriate drug in the prescribed dose are excluded from the study.

In contrast, a pragmatic trial of medical versus surgical treatment for menorrhagia will include all women with a subjective complaint of heavy menstrual loss. Women randomised to drug treatment who find the intervention unacceptable and elect for surgery do not face disqualification from the trial. In a trial evaluating antenatal care, pregnant women may choose to trade in their allocated treatment (reduced antenatal care) for the alternative intervention (routine antenatal care) and still remain in the trial. This somewhat relaxed policy is justified on the grounds that women's decisions to reject their allocated treatment are likely to reflect real-life situations and can actually be interpreted as a measure of dissatisfaction.

There are other differences between the two types of trials. Blinding is more likely to be used in an explanatory trial. Participants in pragmatic trials may also be blinded but this is neither feasible (for example, surgical versus medical treatments for urinary incontinence or planned caesarean section versus planned vaginal birth in breech presentation) nor desirable in all circumstances. There is also less of a compulsion to use a placebo in pragmatic drug trials, as the objective is to compare the new intervention with the 'gold standard' or best of the existing treatments. The outcome in a pragmatic trial such as one comparing oral clomifene citrate (a drug treatment) versus expectant management (no treatment) in unexplained infertility assesses the total difference between the interventions including the effect of the treatment as well as the associated placebo effect.[8] A similar situation occurs in comparison of hospital-based versus primary care-based antenatal care.

Trial design

Two-arm parallel group

A two-arm parallel group is the simplest and most common trial design involving a comparison between two groups; that is, an experimental versus a control group.

Multiple-arm parallel group

A trial may have more than two arms; for example, intrauterine insemination (IUI) versus ovarian stimulation + intrauterine insemination (OS/IUI) compared with *in vitro* fertilisation (IVF) for the treatment of unexplained infertility.[9] Another example would be a trial on induction of labour comparing titrated oral misoprostol, Foley catheter + titrated oral misoprostol with vaginal dinoprostone.[10] Multi-arm trials have specific statistical issues that require consideration at the design and analysis stages. Such trials may have varying power to show clinical differences between any two arms.

Crossover

In crossover trials, women are randomly allocated to receive one of the treatments first followed by the other. As women act as their own controls, this reduces the sample size for the trial. Often, a 'washout period' is introduced between the two interventions to reduce the risk of contamination (the effect of the first intervention being carried over to the second intervention). This design is more appropriate for medical treatments of chronic conditions such as premenstrual syndrome or sexual function than for conditions where the outcome (for example, live birth in infertility trials or death in oncology trials) takes the participant out of the trial.

Factorial

Factorial designs are considered to be efficient, as they can address two research questions within the context of a single trial. The simplest is a 'two by two' factorial design, an example of which is described in Figure 8.1. Women with unexplained infertility are randomised into four groups to receive either no treatment, clomifene alone, IUI alone or clomifene and insemination treatment.

This design enables two clinical questions to be addressed within a single trial, provided that the two interventions do not interact with one another (for example, the effect of clomifene is unchanged by the concomitant use of IUI and vice versa). In this case, the effect of IUI can be assessed by comparing groups C and D with A and B, while the effect of clomifene can be evaluated by comparing B and D versus A and C. However, if the effect of IUI is influenced by the presence of clomifene, the analysis will lose power. One systematic review concluded that transparent reporting is required to ensure accurate interpretation of factorial trials.[11]

Clomifene	Intrauterine insemination (IUI)	
	No	Yes
No	No treatment *Group A*	IUI *Group C*
Yes	Clomifene *Group B*	Clomifene and IUI *Group D*

Figure 8.1 Factorial design in a fertility trial

Cluster randomised trial

Some interventions in gynaecology and infertility are not targeted at individual patients but at groups of patients, such as general practices or hospitals. This can occur, for example, where the intervention is an information package for the management of menorrhagia in primary care[12] or a clinical guideline for the management of infertility.[13] In these studies, randomising individuals to receive a particular intervention would have introduced contamination, as GPs would be expected to manage both study (information leaflet, clinical guidelines) and control patients. This could potentially underestimate the true effectiveness of the intervention. Thus, clusters of patients (general practices) are randomly allocated to receive intervention (for example, information leaflets, clinical guidelines) or to the control group.

Measurements from individuals within the same cluster will be correlated to one another in a cluster randomisation trial. The extent of the correlation is measured by the intracluster correlation coefficient.[14] This has important implications for the design (for example, sample size), conduct (for example, informed consent), analysis and reporting. When determining the number of patients required, adjustment should be made for the degree of variation within a cluster. This may require the sample size to be inflated by a factor which adjusts for the intracluster correlation coefficient.

Quasi-randomised trials

Quasi-randomised trials are controlled experimental studies where treatment allocation is performed on the basis of odd or even patient unit numbers or days of the week when the patients are recruited. Although this design of treatment allocation affords an element of chance, it cannot be considered to be genuine randomisation. Loss of allocation concealment can lead to deliberate exclusion of some patients. This, in turn, can exaggerate treatment effects.

Patient preference trial

A potential problem in some randomised trials arises when patients or their clinicians refuse randomisation on grounds of strong treatment preferences. Exclusion of these patients may affect the ability to generalise the results, as participants may not be representative. Recruitment of these patients may introduce substantial bias, especially since it is impossible to blind them. In addition, compliance and satisfaction may be higher with the preferred intervention.[15] Where the principal outcome is satisfaction with care, the influence of patient preference can be substantial. The actual effect size will lie between the minimum and maximum values derived from the randomised and the preference arms respectively.[16]

The size of a total partially randomised patient preference cohort will need to be much larger than for a conventional randomised controlled trial. As already mentioned, the size of the randomised cohort needs to be the same as in a conventional trial. In addition, the size of the non-randomised prefer-ence arms needs to be similar. This will add to the cost and duration of the proposed trial. The evidence to support the use of partially randomised patient preference trials compared with conventional randomised trials is limited. Data generated by Cooper *et al.*[17] suggest that the extra cost and complexity of partially randomised patient preference trials were not justified in the context of medical versus surgical treatment of menorrhagia.

Equivalence trials

In some circumstances, the aim is often to show that one treatment is as effec-tive (equivalent) or no less effective (non-inferior) as another. The methodol-ogy for equivalence trials differs to that of superiority trials in design, analysis and interpretation. In designing equivalence trials, attention must be given to defining an equivalence margin, or the difference that would be considered to be 'clinically insignificant'.[18] By definition, this will be smaller than a clinically worthwhile difference, as defined in a superiority trial. Therefore, larger sample sizes are necessary to demonstrate equivalence. The role of conven-tional statistical testing is limited in the analysis of equivalence trials and interpretation of results should be conducted through the use of confidence intervals in relation to the predefined equivalence margin.[19] Statistical signifi-cance is demonstrated if the upper and lower limits of the 95% confidence interval do not cross the equivalence margin.[19]

Bayesian trials

Where trials target interventions in rare conditions where large sample sizes are difficult to achieve, Bayesian methods using all available data may be helpful in determining probabilities. 'Prior' beliefs or expectations about a particular treatment are first determined. The purpose of the trial then is to alter that belief according to the strength of the evidence. Trial data are then analysed as they become available and combined with the amended clinical prior belief or 'posterior distribution' to calculate the probabilities of differ-ent sizes of treatment effects.[20] The general principle is that any decision based on a posterior belief, including data from a randomised trial, is preferable to a decision based on a prior belief alone.

Performing a clinical trial

Systematic review

An essential element of the pre-trial work-up is a systematic review of the lit-erature. This enables the researcher to define the clinical question in the light of previous work and establishes the need for a trial. Information about previ-ous trials, including methodological issues, quality of outcome measures used and duration of follow-up, is useful in planning the study design.

Defining the study population

Identification of an appropriate study population is vital. Disagreement about the definition of a particular condition can lead to dismissal of the conclusions of a trial as irrelevant. For example, the conventional textbook definition of menorrhagia (menstrual blood loss greater than 80 ml) may be unhelpful in defining a study population for a trial of interventions for heavy menstrual bleeding. As menstrual loss is not routinely measured in clinical practice, a pragmatic approach might be to include all women with a subjective complaint of heavy menstrual blood loss. Purists will argue that efficacy of treatments for menorrhagia cannot be evaluated accurately in the absence of patients with 'genuine' pathology. However, the results of trials using rigorous inclusion criteria may not be relevant to the majority of clinics where women are treated on the basis of their subjective symptoms. It is often difficult to define inclusion criteria that are acceptable to all clinicians. For example, agreement on what constitutes a 'short cervix' or 'threatened preterm labour' may be difficult to reach in the context of trials evaluating 'prophylactic' cervical suture or tocolysis. In this situation, it may be helpful to adopt a pragmatic attitude and allow clinicians to use their own clinical judgement to arrive at a diagnosis. This will also increase the ability to generalise the results of such a trial. Explicit description of the eligibility criteria allows the readers to draw their own conclusions regarding the applicability of the data to their own specific contexts. Those performing secondary research can also use these data to assess clinical heterogeneity between trials.

It is particularly important that appropriate steps are taken in order to ensure that the participants are representative of the total eligible population. It may be useful to monitor refusals in order to document whether participants differ substantially from non-participants.

Interventions

Due to its unique mix of medical and surgical treatments, trials in obstetrics and gynaecology offer a number of diverse interventions. Some examples are shown in Table 8.2.

Defining outcomes

For any trial, it is crucial to have a clear research question; that is an initial hypothesis and a clinically relevant primary outcome on which the power calculation is based. Outcomes of choice include those that are purely clinical, patient-centred or economic. The precise nature of the primary and secondary outcomes will depend on the type of trial and its clinical context. This may involve different levels of observation and analysis, incorporating the individual, the family and the community.[21]

Table 8.2 Types of intervention subjected to clinical trials in obstetrics and gynaecology

Intervention	Examples of trials
Packages of care	Use of alternative information packages in use in general practice for treatment and referral in menorrhagia Hospital-based antenatal care versus community-based care
Surgical techniques	Transvaginal tape versus colposuspension for urinary incontinence Hysterectomy versus endometrial resection for menorrhagia Single versus double layer uterine closure for caesarean section
Drug trial	Placebo versus tranexamic acid for menorrhagia Paclitaxel versus carboplatin in ovarian cancer Misoprostol versus dinoprostone gel for induction of labour
Comparison of different treatment modalities	Medical versus surgical termination of pregnancy Levonorgestrel-releasing intrauterine system versus endometrial ablation for menorrhagia Planned caesarean section versus planned vaginal birth in twin gestation/breech presentation
Laboratory techniques	Conventional *in vitro* fertilisation (IVF) versus intracytoplasmic sperm injection Alternative methods of cryopreservation of human embryos in IVF Fluorescence *in situ* hybridisation versus polymerase chain reaction in diagnosis
Place of care	Outpatient versus inpatient endometrial ablation Home versus hospital birth
Investigations	Effectiveness of methods of screening for *Chlamydia trachomatis* The postcoital test in the diagnosis of infertility Group B streptococcus screening in pregnancy Cervical length screening in prediction of preterm labour

Clinical outcomes

Clinical outcomes are essential components of any clinical trial. These are the tools that measure whether the intervention cures or alleviates a certain pathological condition. Generally speaking, outcomes which represent critical events such as live births, deaths and repeat surgery are often more meaningful than outcomes involving measurements of laboratory parameters. In obstetrics, the most meaningful outcomes include perinatal morbidity and mortality rather than duration of labour, time required for induction and birth weight. For example, the proportion of women requiring blood transfusion after hysterectomy is a more clinically relevant outcome than the volume of blood (in millilitres) lost during the procedure. In reproductive medicine, many clinical trials have tended to choose surrogate markers such as number of oocytes retrieved as the primary outcome rather than live birth or pregnancy. The use of a surrogate endpoint can have the effect of reducing the length of a trial and the number of participants required. To detect a difference of 10% in live birth rate, from 30% to 40%, would require a minimum of 477 women in each group, assuming 90% power and 5% significance. However, to detect a difference of one-third of a standard deviation in the number of oocytes retrieved would require a minimum of 191 women per treatment group. When designing clinical trials the aim should be to choose primary outcomes that are clinically meaningful. However, use of surrogate endpoints can reduce the sample size, recruiting time and costs. Where surrogate endpoints are to be adopted in a clinical trial, the effect of the intervention on the surrogate must be highly predictive of the effect on the clinical endpoint.[22]

Explanatory trials usually rely on a single clinical or laboratory outcome. Examples include; menstrual blood loss in millilitres in a trial comparing drug treatments for menorrhagia or induction delivery interval in minutes in a trial on induction of labour.

Pragmatic trials usually require the evaluation of more than one outcome measure in order to inform a clinical decision about the effectiveness, risks, costs and acceptability of an intervention. For example, in surgical trials of menorrhagia, outcomes should include one or more of satisfaction with treatment, menstrual flow, pain, premenstrual syndrome and period of recovery. Trials on expectant management of mild dyskaryosis should include patient attitudes to repeat follow-ups and the proportion of those unwilling to attend follow-up, together with other clinical outcomes such as progression of cervical intraepithelial neoplasia.

Quality of life

Quality of life is a complex concept comprising physical, emotional and other dimensions, which is now accepted as an important outcome in clinical trials.[23] Most commonly used questionnaires not only assess the detailed aspects of quality of life but also provide a summary score for overall health status.[24] Generic measures such as a short-form health survey (SF-36)[25] broadly assess physical, mental and emotional health and can be used to compare conditions and treatments. Although the number of such instruments in current use is rapidly increasing, there is a remarkable level of consistency between them.[23]

A number of condition-specific tools, which can be used either independently or to supplement generic measures, have been developed.[26] Examples include the King's College Questionnaire for Urinary Incontinence[27] and the

Menstrual Distress questionnaire,[28] the Endometriosis Health Profile-30 and the Menopause Rating Scale.[29,30]

Meanwhile, simple global questions on self-reported health or quality of life continue to be useful as prognostic measures for stratification of treatment allocation and as important outcome measures alongside purely clinical outcomes.

Patient satisfaction

There continues to be some disagreement about the mechanisms that produce satisfaction. 'Satisfaction' itself, which has been defined as an 'evaluation based on the fulfilment of expectations',[31] is thought to reflect the sum total of a number of patient-related factors, including expectations, characteristics and psychosocial determinants.[32] Over the past few years, patient satisfaction has become increasingly accepted as a measure of quality in health services and a valid outcome in randomised clinical trials.[33] The particular strength of using satisfaction as an outcome is obvious in certain gynaecological trials, such as those used for menorrhagia or incontinence where not only the interventions (ablation versus hysterectomy or surgery versus physiotherapy) but also the clinical outcomes may be dissimilar. Comparatively, in an obstetric trial comparing caesarean section versus vaginal birth, the importance of including satisfaction as an outcome is clear. However, the routine use of satisfaction as an outcome has its limitations and has been criticised on theoretical and methodological grounds.[34]

Economic evaluation

Pragmatic clinical trials are the standard approach not only for evaluating interventions but also for comparing costs.[35] The costs of treatments are usually estimated using information about the quantities of the resources used. For example, the resources used for hysterectomy include the staff time involved, the consumables used and the length of the subsequent inpatient stay. A trial of continuous electronic monitoring in labour would include costs of staff time as well as the extra interventions (for example, fetal blood sampling and operative deliveries) triggered by the intervention. There may be a need to adopt a societal perspective and include costs to women and their carers. Carrying out an economic evaluation alongside a randomised trial allows detailed information to be collected about the quantities used by each patient in the study.

Power and sample size calculations

Power is the probability that a study of a given size will detect as statistically significant a real difference of a given magnitude.[36] Before embarking on any clinical trial, due consideration should be given to ensure that the study will have adequate power (usually 80% or 90%). If the statistical power is low, the results of the trial will be questionable as the numbers may have been too small to detect genuine differences. In general, a clinically worthwhile difference in the primary outcome should be identified as the point of reference for a sample size calculation. For example, a 20% difference in satisfaction rate between two forms of treatments for incontinence may be considered to be clinically important. Conversely, against a background of low livebirth rates, a difference of 5–10% may be enough to change clinical practice in an infertility trial, as could a small difference in uterine hyperstimulation rates caused by agents used to induce labour.

In determining the sample size, attention should also be paid to the possibility of sample attrition and the need for any future subgroup analysis. For example, in trials of termination of pregnancy, a high non-response to follow-up should be anticipated and the sample size inflated accordingly.[37] Subgroup analyses should be identified in advance and, in general, it should be perceived as a hypothesis-generating exercise. Trials with small sample sizes have a high risk of failing to demonstrate a real difference (type II error). This has often been the case in gynaecological trials.[38] At the same time, aiming for unrealistically large sample sizes is counterproductive and possibly unethical if it means that a trial is abandoned owing to failure of recruitment.

Randomisation

Randomisation involves allocating participants to groups such that individual characteristics do not influence the nature of the intervention. Any difference in outcome is therefore attributable to the treatment alone. Random allocation does not guarantee that the groups will be identical but it does ensure that any differences between them are due to chance alone.

While the simplest method of randomisation is tossing a coin, in practice this is not an accepted method of treatment allocation. The main reason for this is the lack of an audit trail that makes it difficult to confirm that the random allocation was performed correctly. The random allocation should be determined in advance, preferably by using random numbers generated by a mathematical process. After the randomisation list has been prepared (by someone who will not be involved in recruitment), it must be concealed before being made available to researchers. Although the process of randomisation can occur at the recruitment point, this is preferably done at long range, by telephone or even the internet. Alternatively, sequentially numbered opaque envelopes can be used. Differences in outcome between treatment groups are considerably larger in trials where allocation concealment is not strictly enforced, as this produces a clear bias.

While simple randomisation techniques will, on average, allocate equal numbers to each arm, groups of different sizes can result. Block randomisation can be used to keep the numbers in each group close at all times. In a trial of two alternative surgical treatments, we might employ stratified randomisation which produces a separate randomisation list for each surgeon (stratum) so that similar numbers of patients receive both treatments. If envelopes are used, this may involve two separate lists of random numbers and two separate piles of sealed envelopes for each surgeon. With stratified randomisation, we must always use blocks to ensure that there is balance of treatments within each stratum. While stratified randomisation can be extended to two or more stratifying variables, there is a practical limit to the number of strata. Stratification by centre is standard practice in multicentre trials.

Other than in very large trials, random allocation may not provide equal distribution of prognostic factors that are major determinants of treatment outcome. Here, it is still possible to achieve balance using minimisation, which is based on the concept that the next patient to enter the trial is allocated to whichever treatment would minimise the overall imbalance between groups at any stage of the trial. For example, age, previous pregnancy and duration of infertility are important prognostic factors for fertility. Minimisation in this context will require a statement about the actual age groups, for example less than 30 years and 30 or older.

Concealment of allocation

The unpredictability of the randomisation process can only be successful if followed by allocation concealment; that is, concealment of the sequence until patients have been assigned to their groups.[39] Awareness of the next treatment allocation could lead to exclusion of certain women based on their prognosis because they would have been allocated to the perceived inappropriate group. Trials that use inadequate or unclear allocation concealment have tended to yield 40% larger estimates of effect compared with those which used adequate concealment.[40–42] Trials with poorly concealed allocation also generated greater heterogeneity in results; that is, the results fluctuated extensively above and below the estimates from better studies.[40]

Blinding

Double blinding seeks to prevent ascertainment bias, protects the sequence after allocation and cannot always be implemented.[43] As in the case with allocation concealment, lack of blinding may lead to exaggeratedly estimated effects of treatment. A survey of trials in gynaecology found that investigators could have used double blinding more often.[43] When used, methods of double blinding were poorly reported and rarely evaluated.

Exclusions

Exclusions can occur because of eventual discovery about ineligibility, deviations from protocol, withdrawals or losses to follow-up. Exclusions before randomisation do not affect the internal validity of the trial but can compromise the ability to generalise from the results. Exclusions after trial entry represent a significant source of bias within a clinical trial, as any dropout over the course of the trial from the initially randomised participants is not likely to be random in nature. The accepted method of primary analysis in all cases is by 'intention to treat'; that is, analysis of patients in the originally assigned groups regardless of any breaches of protocol.[1] This can prove unnerving for clinicians, especially in the context of surgical trials. For example, in a trial comparing hysterectomy versus endometrial ablation, many clinicians would argue against analysis of amenorrhoea rates by intention to treat. It may be perceived that inclusion of women who had actually undergone hysterectomy in the ablation group would lead to an overestimation of amenorrhoea rates. The advantage of randomisation is entirely lost when investigators exclude participants and in effect present a non-randomised comparison as the primary result; that is, similar to a cohort study. Exclusions of participants can lead to misleading results.[44]

Follow-up

The precise duration of follow-up will depend on the nature of the trial. For menorrhagia trials, 80% of re-treatments occur within 2 years, making this an acceptable duration for follow-up in the first instance. A prolonged period of follow-up of up to 5 years would be ideal, as many women could expect the effects of their treatment to wane over time and for long-term complications of therapy to surface. This would appear to be equally true for urogynaecology trials. For termination of pregnancy, follow-up has to be kept short, as many women may not wish to be contacted at a remote period. For hormone replacement therapy trials seeking to address crucial outcomes such as rates of fracture, cardiovascular disease or Alzheimer's disease, follow-up may need to be extended to tens of years. In obstetric trials, children may need to be followed-up for a number of years to fully evaluate long-term effects of fetal and perinatal interventions.

Data collection

Data in a trial are usually collected from sources such as case notes, local clinic databases and patient questionnaires. Occasionally, interviews may be used to explore areas that are not capable of being probed adequately with questionnaires. General practitioners and local and national databases may also be accessed to obtain clinical information such as re-treatment rates or serious complications about patients who are lost to follow-up.

Data analysis

Data analysis is an important aspect of the trial and errors here can lead to significant bias. As mentioned above, analysis should be by intention to treat. Each woman should be analysed as though she had received the intervention to which she had been randomised. This minimises any bias due to non-random removal of participants from the trial. The exception is explanatory trials, usually phase I and II drug trials, where strict rules of exclusion for protocol violation apply. Occasionally, it may be important from a clinical point of view to perform a separate analysis by treatment received or by design (for example, equivalence trials). This analysis should be clearly described as such and should be used to assess the primary outcome. Intention to treat can cause much consternation among clinicians, particularly in surgical trials where some outcomes may seem absurd, for example continuing menstrual blood loss in women allocated to hysterectomy who did not undergo the operation but were analysed by intention to treat. A data analysis plan should be defined in advance, identifying the statistical analysis to be applied to the data. Infertility trials have potential for 'unit of analysis' error and in a review of 39 trials in this area, this error was identified in 32 (82%) of studies.[38] Using live birth/couple as the primary outcome, with randomisation and analysis at the couple level, will protect studies from 'unit of analysis' errors.

Presenting results

Analysis should follow the data analysis plan as set out in the protocol and the CONSORT[45] recommendations should be observed. Particularly helpful is a trial chart which sets out in an explicit manner any exclusions or loss to follow-up. Results of subgroup analyses should be treated with caution and used mainly as hypothesis-generating exercises in most modest-sized trials. There should be a conscious attempt to limit discussion to the results generated by the trial and avoid speculation.

Ethics of trials

The scientific rationale for conducting trials is collective equipoise. Clinicians need to be genuinely uncertain about the best treatment. In such a clinical situation, there should be no conflict between the interests of those participating in a trial and those who stand to gain in the future. The important issue is that participants are also in personal equipoise and give informed consent.

For all clinical trials, it is sensible from an ethical and financial point of view to have clear stopping rules as part of the original study design. An independent data monitoring committee should be available to review the results of interim analyses. Early stopping should only occur under pre-planned well-specified circumstances, such as a marked superiority or toxicity of one arm of the study that is greater than that originally hypothesised.

Research governance

All randomised trials should be conducted in accordance with principles of good clinical practice. Although at the moment it is only the conduct of drug trials which is governed by legislation,[46] it is important that all clinical trials are performed to a high standard and in accordance with the principles of research governance.

Conclusion

Trials form the fundamental basis of evidence-based medicine. Variation in the quality of individual trials influences the reliability of the data on which much of modern clinical decision-making is based. While the evidence base is more secure in obstetrics owing to the presence of a number of large definitive trials, the situation in gynaecology is less satisfactory, particularly for surgical interventions. Understanding the language of trials is important for researchers and clinicians alike if advances in clinical care are to happen.

References

1. Pocock SJ. *Clinical Trials: A Practical Approach*. Chichester: Wiley; 1983.
2. El-Refaey H, Rajasekar D, Abdalla M, Calder L, Templeton A. Induction of abortion with Mifepristone (RU 486) and oral or vaginal Misoprostol. *N Engl J Med* 1995;332:983–7.
3. Goodwin TM, Valenzuela GJ, Silva H, Creasy G. Dose ranging study of the oxytocin antagonist atosiban in the treatment of preterm labour. Atosiban Study Group. *Obstet Gynecol* 1996;88:331–6.
4. Collaborative Eclampsia Trial Group. Which anti-convulsant for women with eclampsia: Evidence from the Collaborative Eclampsia Trial. *Lancet* 1995;345:1455–63.
5. CLASP Collaborative Group. Low dose aspirin in pregnancy and early childhood development follow-up of the collaborative low dose aspirin study in pregnancy. *Br J Obstet Gynaecol* 1994;102:861–8.
6. Hannah, ME, Whyte H, Hannah WJ, Hewson S, Amankwah K, Cheng M, *et al.* Term Breech Trial Collaborative Group. Maternal outcomes at 2 years after planned caesarean section versus planned vaginal birth for breech presentation at term: The International Randomized Term Breech Trial. *Am J Obstet Gynecol* 2004;191:917–27.
7. Whyte H, Hannah ME, Saigal S, Hannah WJ, Hewson S, Amankwah K, *et al.* Term Breech Trial Collaborative Group. Outcomes of children at 2 years after planned caesarean birth versus planned vaginal birth for breech presentation at term: The International Randomized Term Breech Trial. *Am J Obstet Gynecol* 2004;191:864–71.
8. Roland M, Torgerson DJ. Understanding controlled trials: what are pragmatic trials? *BMJ* 1998;316:285.
9. Goverde AJ, McDonnell J, Vermeiden JPW, Schats R, Rutten FFH, Schoemaker J. Intrauterine insemination or in-vitro fertilisation in idiopathic subfertility and male subfertility: a randomised trial and cost-effectiveness analysis. *Lancet* 2000;355:3–18.
10. Matonhodze BB, Hofmeyr GJ, Levin J. Labour induction at term – a randomised trial comparing Foley catheter plus titrated oral misoprostol solution, titrated oral misoprostol alone, and dinoprostone. *S Afr Med J* 2003;93:375–9.
11. McAlister FA, Strauss SE, Sackett DL, Altman DG. Analysis and reporting of factorial trials. *JAMA* 2003;289:2545–53.
12. Fender GRK, Prentice A, Gorst T, Nixon RM, Duffy SW, Day NE, *et al.* Randomised controlled trial of educational package on management of menor-

rhagia in primary care: the Anglia menorrhagia education study. *BMJ* 1999;318:1246–50.

13. Morrison J, Carroll L, Twaddle S, Cameron I, Grimshaw J, Leyland A, *et al.* Pragmatic randomised controlled trial to evaluate guidelines for the management of infertility across the primary care–secondary care interface. *BMJ* 2001;322:1–7.

14. Kerry SM, Bland JM. The intracluster correlation coefficient in cluster randomisation. *BMJ* 1998;316:1455.

15. Torgerson D, Sibbald B. Understanding clinical trials: what is a patient preference trial? *BMJ* 1998;316:360.

16. Brocklehurst P. Partially randomised patient preference trials. *Br J Obstet Gynaecol* 1997;104:1332–5.

17. Cooper KG, Parkin DE, Garret AM, Grant AM. A randomised comparison of medical and hysteroscopic management in women consulting a gynaecologist for treatment of heavy menstrual loss. *Br J Obstet Gynaecol* 1997;104:1360–6.

18. Piaggio G, Pinol APY. Use of the equivalence approach in reproductive health clinical trials. *Stat Med* 2001;20:3571–87.

19. Jones B, Jarvis P, Lewis JA, Ebbutt AF. Trials to assess equivalence: the importance of rigorous methods. *BMJ* 1996;313:36–9.

20. Lilford RJ, Thornton JG, Braunholtz D. Clinical trials and rare diseases: a way out of a conundrum. *BMJ* 1995;311:1621–5.

21. Roland M, Torgerson DJ. Understanding controlled trials: what outcomes should be measured? *BMJ* 1998;317:1075–80.

22. Fleming TR, DeMets DL. Surrogate endpoints in clinical trials: are we being misled? *Ann Intern Med* 1996;125:605–13.

23. Patrick DL, Bergner M. Measurement of health status in the 1990s. *Annu Rev Public Health* 1990;11:165–83.

24. Fayers PM, Sprangers MA. Understanding self-rated health. *Lancet* 2002;359:187–8.

25. Ware JE, Sherbourne CD. The MOS 36-item short form health survey (SF-36). Conceptual framework and item selection. *Med Care* 1992;30:473–83.

26. Guyatt GH, Bombardier C, Tugwell PX. Measuring disease specific quality of life in clinical trials. *Can Med Assoc J* 1986;134:889–95.

27. Kelleher CJ, Cardozo LD, Khullar V, Salvatore S. A new questionnaire to assess the quality of life of urinary incontinent women. *Br J Obstet Gynaecol* 1997;104:1374–9.

28. Moos RH. Typology of menstrual cycle symptoms. *Am J Obstet Gynecol* 1969;103:390–402.

29. Jones G, Kennedy S, Barnard A, Wong J, Jenkinson C. Development of an endometriosis quality-of-life instrument: The Endometriosis Health Profile-30. *Obstet Gynecol* 2001;98:258–64.

30. Schneider HP, Heinemann LA, Rosemeier HP, Potthoff P, Behre HM. The Menopause Rating Scale (MRS): comparison with Kupperman index and quality-of-life scale SF-36. *Climacteric* 2000;3:50–8.

31. Williams B. Patient satisfaction: a valid concept? *Soc Sci Med* 1994;38:509–16.

32. Sitzia J, Wood N. Patient satisfaction: a review of issues and concepts. *Soc Sci Med* 1997;45:1829–43.

33. Bury M. Doctors, patients and interactions in health care. In: Bury M, editor. *Health and Illness in a Changing Society*. London: Routledge; 1997. p. 77–109.

34. Williams B, Coyle J, Healy D. The meaning of patient satisfaction: an explanation of high reported levels. *Soc Sci Med* 1998;47:1351–9.

35. Drummond MF, Davies L. Economic analysis alongside clinical trials. Revisiting the methodological issues. *Int J Technol Assess Health Care* 1991;7:561–73.

36. Altman DG. *Practical Statistics for Medical Research*. London: Chapman and Hall; 1991.

37. Ashok PW, Kidd A, Flett GM, Fitzmaurice A, Graham W, Templeton A. A randomised comparison of medical abortion and surgical vacuum aspiration at 10–13 weeks gestation. *Hum Reprod* 2002;17:92–8.

38. Vail A, Gardner E. Common statistical errors in the design and analysis of subfertility trials. *Hum Reprod* 2003;18:1000–4.

39. Schulz KF, Grimes DA. Generation of allocation sequences in randomised trials: chance not choice. *Lancet* 2002;359:515–19.

40. Schulz KF, Chalmers I, Hayes RJ, Altman DG. Empirical evidence of bias: dimensions of methodological quality associated with estimates of treatment effects in controlled trials. *JAMA* 1995;273:408–12.

41. Moher D, Pham B, Jones A, Cook DJ, Jadad AR, Moher M, *et al.* Does quality of reports of randomised trials affect estimates of intervention efficacy reported in meta-analysis. *Lancet* 1998;352:609–13.

42. Juni P, Altman D, Egger M. Assessing quality of controlled trials. *BMJ* 2001;323:42–6.

43. Schulz KF, Grimes DA, Altman DG, Hayes RJ. Blinding and exclusions after allocation in randomised controlled trials: survey of published parallel group trials in obstetrics and gynaecology. *BMJ* 1996;312:742–7.

44. Schulz KF, Grimes DA. Sample size slippages in randomised trials: exclusions and the lost and wayward. *Lancet* 2002;359:781–5.

45. Moher D, Schultz KF, Altman DG. The CONSORT statement: revised recommendations for improving the quality of reports of parallel-group randomised trials. *Lancet* 2001;357:1191–4.

46. EU Clinical Trials Directive, Medicines for Human Use (Clinical Trials) Regulations 2004. Directive 2001/20/EC [www.mhra.gov.uk/home/idcplg? IdcService= SS_ GET_PAGE&nodeId=716].

9

Animal research

Fiona Broughton Pipkin

'... not in any way to be enterprised, nor taken in hand, unadvisedly,
lightly or wantonly.'
Solemnisation of Matrimony, The Book of Common Prayer

The use of living animals in scientific procedures is highly contentious. In this chapter, I shall not consider work undertaken to comply with legislation, for example that relating to regulatory toxicology, but will concentrate entirely on biomedical research. Questions about ethics and scientific utility must be asked before any such work is undertaken. Absolutely central to the ethical dimension is the cost–benefit equation. This is because, as distinct from work involving human subjects, there can be no consent by the animal to participation in the research. The individual animal will not benefit from any procedure, as may be the case in human clinical trials, nor will it be aware of its contribution to increasing the sum of knowledge. Its own species may benefit where findings have implications for veterinary medicine but, for our purposes, this is serendipity and not a primary objective. The animal thus bears all the physiological cost in terms of pain, suffering, distress or lasting harm.

Biomedical research is a team activity. No matter how high your clinical standing and technical proficiency, good research requires active input from a range of experts with competencies you are unlikely to have. While in some cases, such as statistics, you may be aware of where to go for advice, this may not be the case in other critical areas, such as the range of available research technologies, the choice of species and experimental model, information management and laboratory animal care including anaesthetic and analgesic practice. If you are considering taking on the role of a project licence holder, all of these areas become your ultimate responsibility.

As with any research, before you start planning it, you must be as sure as you can be that the answer to the question is worth having. This is the 'benefit' aspect of the cost–benefit equation. As in human-based research, it is a good idea to write down a formal list of benefits, rather than having a woolly idea at the back of your head. Be aware that although potential healthcare benefits are obvious legitimate benefits, from a professional and ethical perspective, personal advancement is not. Remember to judge the potential benefits only on the nature and utility of the new information and insights that will be generated rather than simply the importance of the field to which the research relates. Are you certain beyond reasonable doubt that the work has not been done before? With online access to Medline and database services, there is no excuse for not knowing – although in some cases these databases will not reference the earliest studies. It is essential for new researchers to talk through the concepts with a colleague experienced in this type of work.

Once you have decided that there are genuine benefits to be obtained and you think that your hypothesis can reasonably be tested in animals, stop and think again. Do you really have to use live animals? Could you achieve your objectives by some other means? Increasing use is being made of isolated cells and cell and tissue cultures to answer questions at the molecular and genetic level. Computer modelling systems are also increasingly being used to model biological processes within the biomedical sciences. A good source of information about such replacement alternatives is FRAME (Fund for the Replacement of Animals in Medical Research), which has published a useful supplement on replacement models.[1] The Universities Federation for Animal Welfare (UFAW) is another source of information.[2] Their two websites identify a variety of publications relating to the reduction, refinement and replacement of animals in medical research. At the other end of the scale, the development of increasingly sophisticated techniques for measuring physiological variables non- or minimally invasively in man, may mean that a question relating to integrated physiology can now be answered in the species in which you are primarily interested. Have you really investigated these possibilities?

If you cannot undertake the work in human volunteers, will data obtained from animals be of use in relation to man? Much is; some is not. In each case, how will you critically evaluate the scope and limitations of extrapolating animal test data to man? For example, the unravelling of the story of lung surfactant and its vital role in the transition to extrauterine life was almost all carried out in the fetal and newborn lamb and rabbit. These data were directly applicable across species and have proved invaluable. The development and daily use of synthetic surfactant in the treatment of very prematurely delivered babies is a clear example of the value of curiosity-driven research generating hypotheses, tested in animals and going on to the development of entirely novel therapeutic measures. Conversely, some aspects of placental physiology in the sheep differ markedly from our own and some aspects of equine reproduction cannot be extrapolated to any other species group.

If you conclude that you must use animals, and that data so obtained will be relevant to your human patients, then consider what is the most suitable species to use. While it is an essential requirement that the chosen species provides meaningful results, faced with a choice of suitable species or stage of development, that believed to have the lowest degree of neurophysiological sensitivity, in terms of capacity to suffer should be selected. It may be possible to use an invertebrate species; our understanding of mammalian nerve conduction has been built on the giant axon of the squid. In considering the use of vertebrates, it is sometimes argued that the life of a rat or mouse is not equivalent to that of a dog, cat or primate – and indeed the current UK legislation reflects this premise. Therefore, if you can use rats or mice, do so. On the other hand, if the question can only properly be answered using a higher species, then justify your choice and use that species. Remember that a careful choice of model should lead to more rapid advances in understanding and should therefore keep the number of animals used to provide meaningful results to the minimum. The use of primates should be avoided if at all possible.

Where would the work be done? In the UK, the use of live vertebrate animals for experimental or other scientific purposes using protocols that may cause pain, suffering, distress or lasting harm is regulated under the Animals (Scientific Procedures) Act 1986, and may only be performed in places holding a Certificate of Designation (see below). Make contact with your university's animal house, talk to those who would be in day-to-day charge of the animals. These people can advise you on the suitability of various species and strains of animal and on aspects of care and accommodation that might affect your experimental results. In addition, remember that the animal care staff may also have the experience to undertake routine dosing and sampling procedures more competently and with less stress to the animals than you. Talk to the veterinary surgeon with responsibility for the animal house. Quite apart from any surgical and experimental skills which may be required, there will be questions of suitable anaesthetic techniques, postoperative care if recovery experiments are to be performed, the determination, recognition and implementation of clinical end-points (including the necessary observation schedules) mandating the humane killing of the animal, regardless of whether the experiment is complete or not, and the final euthanasia of the animal.

Are your clinical commitments such that you can in fact 'ringfence' the amount of time required for the work, which is likely to be more than you think? Remember that you should be checking on the condition of all animals at least daily and should be available if the clinical condition of the animals requires more intensive monitoring. If you cannot unequivocally answer 'Yes', then you should obtain funding for a co-worker, whose primary responsibility is to the animal work. Attempting to squeeze experimental work into slots in a demanding clinical schedule all too often results in poorly conducted or unfinished studies, the consequent waste of animals' lives and little of benefit added to our collective knowledge.

Experiments must be designed in association with a statistician, to ensure not only that the minimum number of animals needed to test the hypothesis is used but also that sufficient animals are used to test it properly. Repeatedly, reviews of published work have highlighted glaring statistical errors calling into question, and in some cases overturning, the published findings. Poor science is unethical and should also be unpublishable. Indeed, the publication of questionable findings does science a disservice.

You should familiarise yourself at an early stage in planning your work with the concept of 'the three Rs' – reduction, refinement, replacement – and try to think it through in the context of that work. 'Refinement' in this context implies the identification and introduction of methods which alleviate or minimise the pain, distress or other adverse effects which may be suffered by experimental animals and/or enhance their general wellbeing. Quite apart from the priorities of the application of ethical and humane principles, it should always be remembered that a stressed animal will not give physiologically useful data. Indeed, few would argue in this context with the general proposition that good animal welfare and good science are inseparable. The Boyd Group is a discussion forum that brings together individuals from responsible animal rights and welfare groups, practising scientists and ethicists and sets up working groups to discuss particular topics in relation to the use of animals in biomedical research seeking areas of consensus. The group has published a useful article on current concepts of refinement in animal use.[3] In addition, the Government has established a National Centre for the 3Rs (NC3Rs: www.nc3rs.org.uk) responsible to ministers at the Office for Science and Technology to develop and promote awareness and use of alternative methods.

The ethical review process

At this stage you will have done your background reading, formulated your hypothesis, thought through the cost–benefit equation, investigated alternatives, chosen your species, decided where the work would be done and designed the experiment. You will have discussed the work with a variety of colleagues. You must now submit your work to your local Animal Care and Use Committee for approval.

The Home Office requires that all designated establishments operate a 'local ethical review process' to support and quality assure animal research that the institution believes can be justified, taking into account all aspects of animal production, care and use. Although the Home Office took care to allow for local flexibility and to require a 'process', in many places this is implemented through committee structures.

Such review must be tailored to meet the needs of the establishment and the aims of the policy. The Animals Procedures Committee, which advises the Government on the workings of the 1986 Act (see below) gave information about five possible models for establishment-based ethical review in its 1995 Report.[4] Either the senior colleague who will be advising on the work or the head technician in your animal house will be able to tell you what the local arrangements and requirements for this committee are. Such committees have various names but their function is to check that you have indeed gone through all the preliminaries with proper care and that the work is ethically acceptable within your community. In addition, you can expect to receive advice, and access to resources, that will improve your plan of work through those involved in this process. Your next step is to acquire the authority under the 1986 Act to perform the work.

The Animals (Scientific Procedures) Act 1986

It is a criminal offence to perform any procedure on a living vertebrate animal (and some cephalopods) for purposes of research unless the programme of work is authorised by a Project Licence, issued by the Home Secretary, and the person undertaking the procedure is the holder of a Personal Licence. It does not matter how experienced a clinician you are, there are no exemptions. Everyone applying for a Personal Licence and/or Project Licence must undergo formal training through an accredited training scheme and be certified as having successfully done so. Consult the head technician in your animal house for details of the requirements and the local arrangements.

You must then fill out a detailed application form for a Personal Licence for permission to undertake the procedures that you yourself will be performing and the species to which they will be applied. Once awarded, the Personal Licence authorises you to undertake only those procedures on those species; if you subsequently discover that you need to use other procedures or species, further formal authorisation must be sought and given, and your licence amended, before they can be used. Be aware that as a personal licence holder you are personally accountable to the Home Office for the welfare of animals on which you have performed regulated procedures. Personal Licences may only be used in conjunction with a Project Licence.

A Project Licence authorises a programme of work, for specified purposes and objectives, which requires the application of specified regulated procedures to animals of specified descriptions at a specified place or places. It is granted by the Home Secretary to the person who assumes overall responsibility for the programme specified in that licence. The Project Licence holder is personally responsible for compliance with the terms and conditions of the licence – and for ensuring compliance by the personal licensees working on the Project Licence. If you are new to work with animals, it is strongly advised that you identify a senior colleague with relevant experience to advise you and collaborate with you. It may be appropriate and possible for you to work initially under a modification of their Project Licence providing it can be amended to incorporate your programme of work. A revised Project Licence form was introduced in December 2004, which includes the provision of a short abstract describing the proposal in lay terms to be displayed in anonymised form at the Home Office website if and when the Project Licence is granted.

Once written, the applications for Project and Personal Licences are sent to the Home Office for authorisation. No work may be undertaken until the licences have been awarded. Although 85% of Project Licence applications are processed within 7 weeks, not all are granted, and more contentious proposals can take many months to consider.

Overseeing the workings of the Act in the university where you work will be an inspector from the Home Office. Inspectors are all either registered medical or veterinary practitioners with higher academic and/or professional qualification and experience of various aspects of biomedical research. Remember when drafting your application that the inspector may have a sound general knowledge of science, but will almost certainly not be a specialist in your field, and draft applications accordingly. Inspectors scrutinise all licence applications, and advise the Home Office on whether and on what terms licence authorities should be granted. Inspectors make both scheduled and unscheduled visits to the university; during the course of the inspections they will certainly see your animals and may wish to speak with you or look at your records. You should arrange to meet your local inspector as soon as you begin to consider doing work with living animals and certainly before you seek funding or begin to complete a licence application. The inspector will be able to advise on administrative procedures for your applications and on such matters as potential local advisors and collaborators (see above). At this preliminary stage you may also be advised on any aspect of the work which is likely to prove contentious and the arguments you will have to muster for the application to be properly considered. It is also helpful for the inspector to be forewarned of the area of work for which an application may be submitted, so that they can undertake any necessary background reading and identify colleagues in the Inspectorate with the most appropriate background to work with them in assessing the application.

Work may only be carried out in a place designated as a scientific establishment by a Certificate issued by the Home Secretary. Indeed, animals may only be held and used in the specific areas within such establishments that have been approved for this purpose. In academic life, the 'Certificate Holder' is almost invariably a senior member of the university's administrative staff, such as the Registrar or Assistant Registrar. The Certificate Holder is responsible for ensuring, through a clear management line, that all work undertaken under the Act is in accordance with it. You are responsible for ensuring that you understand this management line and comply with its requirements.

You are legally required to submit a return of all work performed under the Act in the preceding calendar year in the early spring of the next year. The legal requirements for record keeping are covered in the training course. These records and laboratory notebooks are, of course, extremely important scientifically and must also be available to the inspector on request at any time.

Informing the public

The UK has both a thriving biomedical research sector and a long, honourable and worldwide reputation for the concern of its population for the wellbeing of animals, whether domesticated or wild. However, a large and increasing proportion of that population is now urban or suburban and only comes in direct contact with living animals under highly artificial circumstances. Its anthropomorphic perceptions of the animal kingdom frequently appear to be based on those of the sentimentalising media and cartoon characters, while biomedical scientists are too often portrayed by the same media as ghouls. In addition, even within the medical profession there is often ignorance about the contributions animal use has made and continues to make to healthcare technologies, including the fact that animal testing is still a mainstay of establishing the safety and efficacy of novel pharmaceuticals to the satisfaction of the relevant regulatory authorities. An industry has grown up which attempts to convince schoolchildren that research using living animals is intrinsically and always unjustifiable. It receives generous funding from several 'animal welfare' charities and provides extensive campaigning material to schools and others. Debate should most certainly be stimulated on the topic, but it must be informed from both sides to be of any value. As doctors and scientists, we have traditionally been more focused on informing our peers rather than informing and engaging with the public. It has been established that the general public is willing to support biomedical research involving animals providing it is justified, properly conducted, causes only the minimum resulting suffering, and is strictly regulated.

No one should undertake research using living animals unless they and their peers are convinced of the value of, and justification for, so doing. Once you have decided that such work is valuable and justified, and begun publishing so that the work is in the public domain, think about agreeing to take part in local debates, whether in a school or college, or on local radio or television. The Research Defence Society will give expert help in preparing for such a role; do make use of them. This gives you the opportunity to explain and justify why such work is necessary, to point out any direct implications of your work for clinical care and to describe the numerous levels of controls that have to be gone through before and during any such work. It is disgraceful that a few violent extremists should have terrorised some research workers to the point where they are unwilling to speak about their work publicly other than at scientific meetings. Such extremists have no place in an educated and thinking society.

Acknowledgement
I am most grateful to Dr Jon Richmond, Head, Animals (Scientific Procedures) Division at the Home Office, for his reading of, and constructive comments on, this chapter.

References
1. Balls M, editor. Alternatives to animal experiments: progress made and challenges ahead. The proceedings of the ECVAM Status Seminar 2002, held on 4–6 June 2002, Ispra, Italy. *Altern Lab Anim* 30;Suppl. 2:1–243 [http://altweb.jhsph.edu/publications/journals/atla/30_sup2/atla30_suppl2-toc.htm].

2. Poole TB, editor. *The UFAW Handbook on the Care and Management of Laboratory Animals.* 7th ed. Oxford: Blackwell Publishing; 1999.
3. Advancing refinement of laboratory animal use. *Lab Anim* 1998;2:137–42.
4. Animal Procedures Committee. *Report of the Animal Procedures Committee for 1995.* London: The Stationery Office Ltd; 1996.

10

Fetal research

Nicholas M Fisk and Keelin O'Donoghue

The problem

The sanctity of the fetal environment provides a formidable barrier to research endeavour. The fetus lies, inaccessible, within the pregnant abdomen, vulnerable to exogenous insults causing teratogenicity, miscarriage and prematurity. Mothers, understandably, regard their babies as 'precious' and ethical constraints preclude all but 'trivial risk' research. Whereas adult medicine advances apace owing to modern technology, fetal medicine lags well behind, denied the progress in knowledge that would accrue from positron emission tomography, nuclear medicine, interventional radiology, metabolic challenge, cardiac catheterisation, direct drug therapy, invasive circulatory monitoring, chronic arterial or venous access and serial tissue biopsy.

The field

The modern subspecialty of fetal medicine owes its origins to two parallel developments, the advent of high-resolution ultrasound and the access to the fetus provided by invasive procedures. In particular, fetal blood sampling allowed biochemical and haematological investigation as well as direct therapy by transfusion. Despite considerable research activity using these tools over the last 15–20 years, many questions remain. In physiological terms, for instance, we do not understand what causes circulatory redistribution (brain sparing) in response to hypoxaemia, while in clinical terms there has to date been only one randomised controlled trial (RCT) published for any invasive fetal therapy.[1]

Fetal medicine, however, is by no means limited to ultrasound and invasive procedures. A glance at the index of any of the mainstream journals in obstetrics and gynaecology reveals that around 50% of published articles deal with the fetus and/or placenta. The 'big three' problems in obstetric practice: preterm labour, growth restriction and pre-eclampsia, are arguably more fetal than maternal, their origins lying with impaired trophoblastic invasion or altered signalling between the fetus and placenta/membranes. Miscarriage also is most commonly attributable to fetal causes, while the immunology of pregnancy, in particular the non-rejection of the fetoplacental allograft, remains a puzzle. Transplacental drug therapy provides two of the few proven successful treatments in obstetrics: corticosteroids to enhance lung maturity and periconceptual folate to prevent neural tube defects. Finally, the genetic revolution resulting from advances in molecular biology, together with the human genome project, will have major impact, not just in prenatal diagnosis and disease susceptibility but also in developing better therapies, particularly drugs, through pharmacogenomics. Although gene therapy has so far been disappointing with little application *in utero*, the advantages of intrauterine stem cell transplantation already obvious in animal models may, in future, render this the preferred approach for genetic manipulation of autologous cells to cure paediatric and even adult disease.

Fetal ethics

Ethics, law and public moral sensitivity vary widely from country to country. In those where termination is proscribed, some types of fetal research may be problematic, not only those involving fetal tissues but also those involving invasive procedures, the predominant indication for which is fetal karyotyping. On the other hand, in such jurisdictions there is instead opportunity for other forms of research not possible elsewhere, such as the prediction of neurological outcome in fetuses with open spina bifida or ventriculomegaly.

This section of the chapter is necessarily parochial, based on UK practice, but its principles are applicable to many other jurisdictions. Fetal research in the UK was governed for many years by the 1989 report of the Polkinghorne Committee entitled, *Code of Practice on the Use of Fetuses and Fetal Material in Research and Treatment*.[2] Since 2004, the Human Tissue Act has provided the national framework for regulating the storage and use of human organs and tissues from the living as well as the removal, storage and use of organs and tissues from the deceased. The Human Tissue Authority (HTA), which came into being on 1 April 2005, has issued Codes of Practice, which lay down the standards now expected of practitioners and is responsible for licensing and regulating establishments using human tissues.

Human Tissue Act

The Human Tissue Act 2004 makes consent the fundamental principle underpinning the lawful retention and use of body parts, organs and tissues from the living or dead. The HTA's Code of Practice on consent clarifies that the Act does not distinguish between fetal tissue and other tissue from the living – 'fetal tissue is regarded as the mother's tissue'. However, the HTA states, 'because of the sensitivity attached to this subject, consent should be obtained for the examination of fetal tissue and for its use for all scheduled purposes, regardless of gestational age. It is considered good practice, that wherever practicable, consent should also be obtained for the use in research of non-fetal products of conception'. Further, the Code states that local research ethics committee approval is always required for the use of fetal tissue and products of conception in research.[3]

The Code of Practice on the removal, storage and disposal of human organs and tissues also states that consent should where possible be obtained for the use of tissue removed from the living for 'research into disorders or the functioning of the human body'. Where this is not possible, it is lawful for material taken from a living person to be stored without consent for research purposes only if the research is ethically approved, the material is anonymised, and the researcher takes all necessary steps not to identify the person from whose body the material has come.[4] Eventual disposal of fetal tissues should be in accordance with guidance given by Appendix B of the HTA Code of Practice.[4] The Royal College of Obstetricians and Gynaecologists (RCOG) has also issued guidelines on the disposal of fetal tissues following pregnancy loss before 24 weeks of gestation.[5]

Live fetuses

Under UK law, the fetus is not considered a person at any gestation and has no independent legal rights before birth. Beneficence-based ethics holds that, in continuing pregnancies, the mother bestows moral status on her fetus and, thus, the obligation to do good rather than harm. It has been argued that the fetus acquires independent moral status (that is, independent of maternal intent) after viability,[6] although this appears overly simplistic in countries such as the UK where the mother can elect to undergo late termination to prevent severe handicap in the child.

As the Human Tissue Act regards fetal tissue as the mother's tissue, the mother must therefore give appropriate consent to research on the living fetus. The Polkinghorne report recommended that research on living fetuses should be treated on principles broadly comparable to those applicable to children and adults, which preclude intervention above minimal risk, except on balance of benefit to the fetus.[2] The stringent ethical principles pertaining to research on children are considered to apply particularly to the fetus.

Dead fetuses

Most fetal tissue for research is derived from terminations. Tissue can be used after spontaneous fetal demise but there are difficulties. These relate not only to the normality and representative nature of specimens, such as after first-trimester miscarriage, but also to postmortem change in the interval from demise till delivery, the latter precluding expression studies and in many cases cytogenetic, immunocytochemical and histological investigation.

Tissue of a fetus *in utero* and that of a fetus *ex utero* (up to 24 weeks of gestation and not born alive) is the woman's tissue and can be treated like other 'residual tissue' following clinical and diagnostic procedures. As such, aborted fetuses fall under the provision of the Human Tissue Act 2004, which sets out requirements for specific consent to the use of human tissue in research. The principle of the Polkinghorne guidelines was that the decisions and actions relating to the process of termination of pregnancy should be separated from the decisions and actions relating to use of the material, and consent should be general, not specific.[2] The first was not practicable for consent involving invasive procedures and the second became increasingly out of alignment with modern standards of consent. Polkinghorne like all predecessors has now been entirely replaced by the HTA guidance on consent. What constitutes appropriate consent in relation to research on aborted fetuses is defined in the Codes of Practice on consent (paragraph 66).[4]

Studies where the mother is asked to consent to additional research procedures during termination, such as transabdominal needling of the extra-embryonic coelom, yolk sac or fetal circulation have been approved on an individual basis by ethics committees.

Other fetally derived tissues
The contents of the uterus other than the fetus (membranes, amniotic fluid and placenta) may be used under these Codes, providing the mother consents to any additional tests and is not under financial inducement. Traditionally, ethical approval has not been considered necessary for research on tissues that would otherwise be discarded but changes in 2001, in both informed consent and patient sensitivity to their 'ownership' of their own tissues makes this essential[7] and a prerequisite for publications in most journals. The HTA Codes of Practice state that local ethics committee approval is always required for the use of products of conception in research.

Clinical research
Like obstetrics in general, fetal research is beset by the problem of numbers: pathological fetuses and pregnancies are rare amid an overwhelming background of normal pregnancies. The importance of paying attention to the power in any study design is emphasised elsewhere in this book; research on fetal abnormalities or survival needs either to be conducted on high-risk groups and referral populations or to be multicentred.

Epidemiology and audit
Audit of practice in individual centres provided much of the early insight into fetal medicine. With computerised databases and increasing caseload in referral centres, reasonable data now exist on the outcome of prenatally diagnosed abnormalities and the frequency of aneuploidy in association with various ultrasonic markers. The latter were largely univariate analyses with single markers, now superseded by multiparameter aneuploidy risks combining serial biochemistry and ultrasound, as reported in the US multicentre First- and Second-Trimester Evaluation of Risk (FASTER) trial[8] and the UK Serum, Urine and Ultrasound Screening Study (SURUSS).[9] Audit of fetal outcome after various anomalies or invasive procedures in individual centres does have a local role in education and maintenance of standards but is unlikely to contribute to the literature unless multicentre or based on large numbers over many years.

Publications from referral centres are necessarily biased by the selected nature of their referral population. Epidemiological studies yield more representative information based on regional or national data. Examples include regional congenital malformation registries, data from the Office for National Statistics on Down syndrome and termination for fetal abnormality, data reported by the newly-established UK Obstetric Surveillance System (UKOSS), perinatal surveillance data reported to the British Paediatric Association and the national perinatal mortality audits from the Confidential Enquiries into Stillbirth and Death in Infancy (CESDI) and more recently, the Confidential Enquiry into Maternal and Child Health (CEMACH).[10–12] The analysis of such data is relatively straightforward; the difficulty lies in instituting a prospective system of uniform reporting with complete ascertainment.

Observational research

Observation comprises the bulk of published research to date in fetal medicine. It has typically involved ultrasound and/or Doppler observations, either longitudinally, to determine pregnancy changes and outcome, or cross-sectional comparisons of normal with abnormal fetuses. The popularity of this type of research stems from its ethical simplicity and the ready availability of clinical material. The longer the subspecialty exists, however, the less original this type of research becomes. Notwithstanding this, observational studies will continue to generate novel data owing to advances in imaging, such as three- and four-dimensional (4-D) scanning, ultra-fast magnetic resonance imaging and advances in Doppler methods, allowing study of increasingly smaller fetal vessels such as the fetal coronary and adrenal arteries. High-quality volume data from 4-D scanning are now used to generate cross-sectional images or make measurements in planes other than those originally scanned, as shown in the examination of the fetal heart by 4-D ultrasound with spatio-temporal image correlation (STIC).[13]

In addition to anomaly and aneuploidy detection, ultrasound and Doppler are increasingly applied to the prediction of preterm labour (transvaginal assessment of cervical length) and pre-eclampsia (uterine artery Doppler) and to characterising inter-twin transfusion in monochorionic twins.[14] Another application of Doppler, examination of the peak systolic velocity in the fetal middle cerebral artery, has almost replaced invasive methods of testing fetal anaemia.

Special consideration needs to be given to comparing groups of fetuses at different gestations. Analysis of covariance can be used to control for gestational age in studies of relatively small numbers but the preferred technique involves expressing variables in gestational independent Z-scores or standard deviations. The construction of a normal or reference range across gestation is complex, requiring attention not only to sufficient numbers but also to the normality of distribution across gestation.[15] As a general rule, 20 patients are required for construction of a longitudinal reference range and 100–200 for a cross-sectional range.

Before reporting abnormal findings, one must be confident of what is normal and here a sound grounding in fetal physiology is advantageous. Much research in this area has been performed by those whose predominant interest lies not in fetal medicine but in ultrasound, often more generally applied to obstetrics and gynaecology. This has perpetuated several misconceptions, such as in relation to the predictive value of fetal breathing movements, which, by definition, are episodic in nature and change markedly in pattern with fetal maturation.

A further difficulty arises when evaluating tests of fetal wellbeing, if these are disclosed to clinicians. A useless test to predict perinatal survival may appear beneficial in such trials, if the treatment instituted is of value; that is, delivery. Alternately, a very useful test will not appear so if the intervention is useless. Once nondisclosure trials have confirmed associations with adverse outcome, the clinical utility of disclosing such information to clinicians should be evaluated in randomised trials. A good example of this is the development of umbilical artery Doppler monitoring in high-risk pregnancies, still the only diagnostic test shown in RCTs to reduce perinatal mortality.

Invasive procedures

The access to the fetus provided by invasive procedures, in particular fetal blood sampling, led to a plethora of observational studies in the late 1980s, which established baseline biochemical, haematological, immunological and endocrinological parameters. This procedure has been in relative decline since the early 1990s,[16] owing to more rapid non-blood karyotyping techniques, polymerase chain reaction (PCR)-based diagnosis in amniotic fluid, better risk estimation from ultrasound findings and Doppler to predict fetal wellbeing, as well as access to fetal DNA in the maternal circulation.[17] Accordingly, many units set up banks of small additional aliquots of fetal blood and other fluids collected routinely with ethical approval at clinically indicated fetal blood and other sampling procedures. Much of the interesting research has already been done, although the discovery of new enzymes, hormones, cytokines and cell types,[18] as well as new conditions, will see this remain a useful resource.

Because fetal blood sampling carries more than a trivial risk to the fetus, it seems unlikely that ethics committees would approve fetal blood sampling for non-therapeutic research purposes alone. Notwithstanding this, a few groups have used fetal blood sampling to investigate preterm labour, one American group arguing that this practice is acceptable provided that the mother is fully informed.[20] On the other hand, therapeutic research involving risky invasive procedures should prove acceptable to ethics committees, provided that there is, on balance, a prospect of more harm than good to the fetal patient.

There are special difficulties with evaluating invasive procedures. Ideally, these should be compared in RCTs with control groups not undergoing an invasive procedure. This creates understandable difficulty with recruitment. For diagnostic procedures, patients are reluctant to accept a chance of randomisation to no diagnostic test, while for invasive therapies such as vesico-amniotic shunting, many parents are keen to do everything possible for their fetus, even if the proposed treatment is experimental. It is worth remembering that there has been only one trial completed to date with randomisation to an invasive versus no procedure.[20] It is almost impossible to envisage women with high-order multiple pregnancies consenting to a randomised trial of multifetal pregnancy reduction versus conservative management.

Most of the diagnostic procedures have thus been evaluated against other invasive procedures: amniocentesis versus chorion villus sampling (CVS), transabdominal versus transcervical CVS. Even here, recruitment difficulties can limit the power of an RCT where patients are allowed to choose their preferred procedure outside randomisation. Given these difficulties, even recent cohort studies concluding that amniocentesis and CVS loss rates have converged over time are unlikely to be confirmed in an RCT. One way around this is to confine offers of a new procedure within the context of an RCT, although to be effective this may require a national approach as happened in Canada with the introduction of CVS.

No matter how attractive, new procedures must always undergo evaluation, because of the possibility that they may be deleterious. An example is the theoretically attractive procedure of early amniocentesis, now shown in several randomised trials to cause talipes and have a higher miscarriage rate than CVS. A further difficulty is deciding at what time in its development a procedure should be subjected to an RCT; too early and the results may mislead owing to inexperience with the technique, too late and there may be recruitment difficulties.

Many of the newer procedures have infrequent indications, such as fetal endoscopy and vascular ablation techniques. For these, evaluation by case series, comparison with historical and then non-randomised controls seems initially acceptable. Nevertheless, there has still been no assessment of efficacy for some rare procedures in use for over 20 years, such as vesico-amniotic shunting. Pooling multicentre experience is one way around this, as is Bayesian analysis of prior belief adjustment, whereby results are expressed in terms of the percentage chance that a treatment is beneficial (that is, 90%) rather than rejected as of no benefit when the P value falls short of conventional significance (that is, $P = 0.25$). RCTs remain the ideal although, as Lilford et al.[21] point out, the numbers are against them, with a population of 12 million pregnancies required for adequate power for a trial of shunting fetuses with pleural effusions.

The RCT demonstrating that fetoscopic laser ablation of placental vascular anastomoses is an effective treatment of twin–twin transfusion syndrome

(TTTS) has revived interest in endoscopic fetal surgery. Minimally invasive fetoscopic surgery is now both feasible and acceptable in terms of safe fetal access and few maternal complications, although it is restricted to experienced operators in a small number of centres. Proponents suggest fetoscopy may allow for new fetal therapies and/or robotic surgery support in more complex therapeutic procedures in the fetus.[22]

Drugs

Fetal medicine as a branch of medical practice uses surprisingly few drugs. Only periconceptual folate to prevent spina bifida, corticosteroids to mature fetal lungs and low-dose aspirin are of proven benefit in RCTs. Any role for other drugs, such as immunoglobulin therapy in alloimmune disease or urso-deoxycholic acid in obstetric cholestasis, remains controversial. Other drugs may harm the fetus, such as long-term use of the tocolytic indomethacin. The mode of drug delivery may also prove problematic, as illustrated by anti-arrhythmic drugs, which, on the one hand cross the placenta poorly, especially in the presence of hydrops, while, on the other hand their direct administration to the fetus necessitates excessively frequent intrauterine procedures. Drug carrier systems, such as liposomes, may in future be used to retard or facilitate transplacental drug passage.[23] Notwithstanding this, research on direct drug injection in the fetus has led to potential clinical uses of opioid analgesia and contrast agents.[24,25]

Although the risk of teratogenicity (remember thalidomide and stilboestrol) provides powerful disincentives to experimentation in this area, such risks are largely confined to the first trimester and then only to a few drugs. Because the Medicines Licensing Act 1968 permits individual doctors to prescribe drugs for unlicensed use on their own responsibility, drug companies with product licenses for non-obstetric drugs with obstetric applications are understandably reluctant to do research in this area. This explains why few drugs are licensed for use in pregnancy, other than those with pregnancy-only application such as tocolytics and uterotonics. Indeed, corticosteroids to enhance lung maturity remain unlicensed for this purpose.[26] This slows research in obstetric therapeutics by preventing drug company funding.

Anyone proposing a trial involving an unlicensed drug or a licensed drug not licensed for that particular purpose in pregnancy (that is, almost all drugs) requires, in addition to ethical approval and institutional sponsorship, Clinical Trial Authorisation (CTA) from the Medicines and Healthcare products Regulatory Authority (MHRA).

Laboratory research
Animal
The advantages are two-fold. Firstly, there are fewer ethical constraints, such that invasive, longitudinal and terminal studies with immediate access to

pathological tissue are feasible. Secondly, robust design controls for the numerous variables that beleaguer clinical studies, so much so that study numbers of six in each group (intervention and control) often yield significant results. The catheterised fetal sheep has proved a popular model, although chronic experiments remain a challenge, despite the relative inertia of the ovine uterus. Because their placentation is different from that in humans, being epitheliochorial and cotyledonary, non-human primate models with their single disc haemochorial placentas are preferred. Their use in all but a few centres has been precluded by cost. Smaller animals are used for studies of new drugs and cellular and gene replacement therapies, while 'knock out' or 'knock in' mice lacking or over-expressing a certain gene increasingly provide useful insights into embryology, developmental biology and tera-togenesis. See Chapter 9 for a full discussion of animal experimentation.

Trophoblast and placenta

The dually-perfused isolated placental lobule, which mimics the fetoplacental and uteroplacental circulations *in vitro*, is commonly used to study placental transfer under experimental conditions. It remains viable for up to a few hours, sufficient for study of bidirectional transport and equilibration. Concerns about how physiological such perfusion is, can be addressed by serial monitoring of perfusion, flow and pressure, pH and acid–base status.[23] The disadvantages of this model are that technical considerations largely limit it to study of the term, thus normal, placenta, not those complicated by growth restriction, pre-eclampsia, infection or hydrops earlier in pregnancy. An alternative is to study transplacental transfer of drugs at fetal blood sam-pling, although this precludes use of radiolabels and is limited to pregnancies with a clinical indication both for drug administration and fetal blood sampling.

Microvillus membrane preparations of syncytiotrophoblast are used to study the mechanism of transfer across the placenta (endocytosis, paracellular channels). Cell lines of trophoblast can be used to study cell signalling and decidual interactions, although there remains concern about the maintenance of a cell's native characteristics following the immortalisation process. These can be transduced with reporters to unravel triggers to gene expression in the placenta. Finally, placental bed biopsies are used in pathological pregnancies, in an attempt to understand the cellular events mediating impaired trophob-last invasion. A major limitation is that these biopsies are obtained months after the primary and secondary waves of trophoblast invasion and as such represent only the burnt-out embers of the disease process.

Fetal stem cells

Stem cells have been isolated at all stages of development from the early devel-oping embryo to the post-reproductive adult organism. However, the fetal environment is unique as it is the only time in ontogeny that there is migration of stem cells in large numbers into different organ compartments. While fetal neural and haemopoietic stem cells have been well characterised, only relatively recently have mesenchymal stem cells from the human fetus been isolated and evaluated.[18,27]

Fetal mesenchymal stem cells are true multipotent stem cells with greater self-renewal and differentiation capacity than their adult counterparts. They circulate in first trimester fetal blood, from where they traffic into the maternal circulation, and can also be detected in amniotic fluid and among trophoblast. Research on fetal mesenchymal stem cells now focuses on potential downstream applications in fetal cellular and gene therapy in utero. Using mesenchymal stem cells in fetal therapy offers the theoretical advantages of avoidance of immune rejection, increased engraftment, and treatment before disease pathology sets in. Candidate diseases for development of *in utero* transplantation using stem cells include osteogenesis imperfecta, enzyme deficiency diseases such as the mucopolysaccharidoses and the muscular dystrophies. While *in utero* transplantation has been attempted in a number of human pregnancies using allogeneic haemopoietic stem cells, most cases resulted in no engraftment of the transplanted cells, with the few documented successes being limited to fetuses with immunodeficiency syndromes. Mesenchymal stem cells are an alternative target and, although already transplanted in one human fetus with osteogenesis imperfecta, remain predominantly under investigation in murine models of genetic disease.[27,28]

Fetal gene therapy is hypothesised as an approach to the management of otherwise incurable disease. Stem cells have considerable utility as targets for gene therapy because they can self renew, thus precluding the need for repeated administration of the gene vector. *Ex vivo* gene therapy uses autologous stem cells, such as mesenchymal stem cells, which are then transduced by an integrating vector and clonally expanded before re-infusion back into the patient.[27,28] Proof of principle for fetal gene therapy has been provided in murine models of disease but concerns about safety and efficacy remain.[29]

Molecular biology

Molecular genetic techniques are no longer the province of molecular biologists and instead are used in virtually all laboratory-based research. Although much work has been done on conventional DNA testing by PCR for inherited disease in the field of prenatal diagnosis, detecting mRNA using reverse transcriptase PCR is integral to determining the expression and regulation of proteins and enzymes in any reproductive tissue, such as hormones and cytokines mediating the onset of labour in membranes and myometrium. With the human genome-mapping project now complete, an increasing number of disease-susceptibility genes are being cloned. Increasingly, these involve minor changes in short tandem repeats and particularly single nucleotide polymorphisms, of which there are over a million present in the human genome. An example may be that for obstetric cholestasis, following which a reverse genetic approach could be used, as it was for cystic fibrosis, to determine the protein basis of this disorder and ideally develop more rational drug therapies. It is also likely that more genes influencing multifactorial conditions will be identified; examples so far include the wild-type methyltetrahydrofolate reductase variant in mothers at risk of neural tube defects and insulin-like growth factor polymorphisms in growth restriction.

Techniques now making a big impact include real-time PCR (Light Cycler™ or Taqman™), which allows contamination-free nucleic acid quantitation without gels and fluorescent sequencing, array-based comparative genomic hybridisation, which allows high-throughput high-resolution analysis of specific chromosomal regions as well as entire chromosomes, and microarray chips, which allow investigation of thousands of polymorphisms or transcripts in a single reaction. Indeed, this has led to the only new antenatal serological test, the use of real-time PCR to determine fetal RhD type noninvasively in the plasma of RhD-negative pregnant women.[30] Comparison gene expression arrays performed on mRNA isolated from amniotic fluid have showed gene expression changes in fetuses of different age, gender and disease status, and hold great potential for identifying unique fetal biomarkers.[17]

Although increasingly research focuses on the transcriptional regulation of gene expression, one must not forget that only about one-third of expressed genes are actually translated into proteins and increasing attention is now being devoted to proteomic techniques with mass spectrometry of SELDI-TOF and MALDI-TOF, which determine protein profiles of previously uncharacterised, particularly low-molecular-weight, proteins. Both techniques have already been applied to the search for apoptotic placental proteins predicting pre-eclampsia as well as the analysis of free fetal DNA in the maternal circulation and the detection of protein biomarkers in Down syndrome fetuses.

Advances in molecular methods now allow prenatal karyotyping on amniotic fluid without the need for culture, with even the more labour intensive multiprobe fluorescence *in situ* hybridisation (FISH) replaced by automated DNA quantitation of short tandem repeats situated near each centromere (QF-PCR). Further, cell free fetal nucleic acids have been detected in amniotic fluid by array-CGH and used to diagnose fetal gender and aneuploidy.[17]

Rare-event techniques should eventually see non-invasive prenatal diagnosis in fetal genetic material in the maternal circulation became a reality, although this will almost certainly now be based on the high levels of circulating trophoblast-derived fetal nucleic acids in maternal plasma, rather than infrequent fetal cells in maternal whole blood.[31] Additional approaches to fetal nucleic acid detection are also under investigation; using different epigenetic modifications in fetal and maternal genes and using SNP allelic ratios in placental RNA. Thus far, only two applications, fetal RhD or Kell blood group typing, and gender determination have been translated into clinical practice, although a promising recent report of placental mRNA polymorphisms showed high sensitivity and specificity for trisomy 21.[32]

Intrauterine events are also being implicated in later onset disease. Although the Barker hypothesis is now well validated, studies of fetomaternal cell trafficking have implicated persistent fetal cells in the maternal bloodstream in the aetiology of autoimmune diseases such as scleroderma and autoimmune thyroiditis. However, fetal cell microchimerism is not always found in association with maternal disease, and as fetomaternal trafficking occurs in all pregnancies, it is now accepted that microchimerism is established in healthy women as well. The persistent fetal cells have tentatively been identified as stem cells, with a potential role in maternal tissue repair during and after pregnancy.[31,33]

Advice

In selecting a hypothesis to test, first pick something achievable within local conditions and facilities. Although it is important to be inspired by your own question, a more pragmatic approach is to look around at the strengths, expertise and clinical material available in your own centre, as these will determine both the feasibility and originality of your project. Remember, research is not difficult but it is a learned exercise; choosing a sympathetic and productive supervisor is a sensible first step. Laboratory research is more controlled and requires a greater time commitment, while clinical research is subject to the vagaries of patient numbers, consent and clinical variation.

Despite the ethical and accessibility problems, fetal research remains a field rich in challenging clinical and scientific questions. The stakes are high, not just because fetal disease is associated with high perinatal morbidity and mortality but also because the intrauterine environment has long-term effects on the health of the offspring. These constraints on fetal research should be seen instead as challenges.

References

1. Senat MV, Deprest J, Boulvain M, Paupe A, Winer N, Ville Y. Endoscopic laser surgery versus serial amnioreduction for severe twin-to-twin transfusion syndrome. *N Engl J Med* 2004;351:136–44.
2. Polkinghorne J. *Review of the Guidance on the Research Use of Fetuses and Fetal Material*. London: HMSO; 1989.
3. Human Tissue Authority. *Code of Practice – Consent*. London: HMSO; 2006.
4. Human Tissue Authority. *Code of Practice – the removal, storage and disposal of human organs and tissues*. London: HMSO; 2006.
5. Royal College of Obstetricians and Gynaecologists. Disposal following pregnancy loss before 24 weeks of gestation. London; 2005.
6. Chervenak F, McCullough L.. Ethics of fetal therapy. In: Fisk NM, Moise KJ Jr, editors. *Fetal Therapy: Invasive and Transplacental*. Cambridge: Cambridge University Press. p. 345–56.

7. Medical Research Council. *Human Tissue and Biological Samples for Use in Research: Operational and Ethical Guidelines*. London: MRC; 2001.

8. Malone FD, Canick JA, Ball RH, Nyberg DA, Comstock CH, Bukowski R, *et al.* First- and Second-Trimester Evaluation of Risk (FASTER) Research Consortium. First-trimester or second-trimester screening, or both, for Down's syndrome. *N Engl J Med* 2005;353:2001–11.

9. Wald NJ, Rodeck C, Hackshaw AK, Walters J, Chitty L, Mackinson AM. First and second trimester antenatal screening for Down's syndrome: the results of the Serum, Urine and Ultrasound Screening Study (SURUSS). *J Med Screen* 2003;10:56–104.

10. Lynn R, Hall SM, The British Paediatric Surveillance Unit. Activities and developments in 1990 and 1991. *Commun Dis Rep CDR Rev* 1992;2:R145–8.

11. Confidential Enquiry into Stillbirths and Deaths in Infancy. *8th Annual Report.* London: Maternal and Child Health Research Consortium; 2001.

12. Confidential Enquiry into Maternal and Child Health. *Stillbirth, Neonatal and Post-neonatal Mortality 2000–2003 England, Wales and Northern Ireland.* London: RCOG Press; 2005.

13. Goncalves LF, Lee W, Espinoza J, Romero R. Examination of the fetal heart by four-dimensional (4D) ultrasound with spatio-temporal image correlation (STIC). *Ultrasound Obstet Gynecol* 2006;27:36–48.

14. Taylor MJ, Denbow ML, Tanawattanacharoen S, Gannon C, Cox PM, Fisk NM. Doppler detection of arterio-arterial anastomoses in monochorionic twins: feasibility and clinical application. *Hum Reprod* 2000;15:1632–6.

15. Royston P. Constructing time-specific reference ranges. *Stat Med* 1991;10:675–90.

16. Fisk NM, Bower S. Fetal blood sampling in retreat. *BMJ* 1993;307:143–4.

17. Maron JL, Bianchi DW. Prenatal diagnosis using cell-free nucleic acids in maternal body fluids: A decade of progress. *Am J Med Genet* 2007;145:5–17.

18. Campagnoli C, Roberts IA, Kumar S, Bennet PR, Bellantuono I, Fisk NM. Identification of mesenchymal stem/progenitor cells in human first trimester fetal blood, liver and bone marrow. *Blood* 2001;98:2396–402.

19. Berry S, Romero R, Gomez R, Ghezzi F, Mazor M, Tolosa JE. Risks and ethical issues of the use of diagnostic cordocentesis in the evaluation of fetuses with preterm labor. Proceedings of the 17th Annual Meeting of the Society of Perinatal Obstetricians, Anaheim, California. *Am J Obstet Gynecol* 1997;176 Suppl 1:S20.

20. Tabor A, Philip J, Madsen M, Bang J, Obel EB, Norgaard-Pederson B. Randomised controlled trial of genetic amniocentesis in 4606 low-risk women. *Lancet* 1986;1: 1287–93.

21. Lilford R, Thornton J, Braunholtz D. Clinical trials and rare diseases: a way out of a conundrum. *BMJ* 1995;311:1621–5.

22. Deprest J, Jani J, Lewi L, Ochsenbein-Kolble N, Cannie M, Done E, *et al.* Fetoscopic surgery: encouraged by clinical experience and boosted by instrument innovation. *Semin Fetal Neonatal Med* 2006;11:398–412.

23. Bajoria R, Oteng-Ntim E, Fisk NM. Transfer and metabolism of thyrotropin releasing hormone across the perfused human term placenta. *J Clin Endocrinol Metab* 1996;81:3476–82.

24. Denbow ML, Welsh AW, Taylor MJ, Blomley MJ, Cosgrove DO, Fisk NM. Twin fetuses: intravascular microbubble US contrast administration: early experience. *Radiology* 2000;214:724–8.

25. Fisk NM, Gitau R, Teixeira JM, Ginnakoulopoulos X, Cameron AD, Glover VA. Effect of direct fetal opioid analgesia on fetal hormonal and haemodynamic stress response to intrauterine needling. *Anesthesiology* 2001;95:823–35.

26. Fisk NM, Shennan AH. Litigation and prescribing drugs for unlicensed indications. *Lancet* 1993;341:1218.

27. O'Donoghue K, Fisk NM. Fetal stem cells. *Best Pract Res Clin Obstet Gynaecol* 2004;18(6):853–75.

28. Chan J, O'Donoghue K, Fisk NM. . Developmental stem cells. In: Studd J, editor. *Progress in Obstetrics and Gynaecology. 17*. London: Churchill Livingstone; 2006.. p. 15–30.

29. Coutelle C, Themis M, Waddington SN, Buckley SM, Gregory LG, Nivsarkar MS, *et al*. Therapy progress and prospects: fetal gene therapy-first proofs of concept-some adverse effects. *Gene Ther* 2005;12:1601–7.

30. Finning KM, Martin PG, Soothill PW, Advent ND. Prediction of fetal D status from maternal plasma: introduction of a new non-invasive fetal RHD genotyping service. *Transfusion* 2002;42:1079–85.

31. Bianchi DWR, Gross E. Lecture. Fetomaternal cell trafficking: a story that begins with prenatal diagnosis and may end with stem cell therapy. *J Pediatr Surg* 2007;42(1):12–18.

32. Lo YM, Tsui NB, Chiu RW, Lau TK, Leung TN, Heung MM, *et al*. Plasma placental RNA allelic ratio permits noninvasive prenatal chromosomal aneuploidy detection. *Nat Med* 2007;13:218–23.

33. O'Donoghue K, Chan J, de la Fuente J, Kennea N, Sandison A, Anderson JR, *et al*. Microchimerism in female bone marrow and bone decades after fetal mesenchymal stem-cell trafficking in pregnancy. *Lancet* 2004;364:179–82.

11

Laboratory research and quality control

D Stephen Charnock-Jones

Many of the principles underlying good-quality laboratory research are also of fundamental importance to non-laboratory-based research. However, when carrying out laboratory-based work, one can readily get distracted by the technology and lose sight of the principles which underlie high-quality research. This is particularly true in fields that make use of modern cellular and molecular techniques where many complex steps are necessary before one actually performs the true experiment.

An essential first step in all research is the formulation of the hypothesis to be tested. Ideally, this should be clear, simple and short. Once your hypothesis has been formulated, the design of the experiments to test this hypothesis should be relatively straightforward. At this point, it is essential to ensure that the experiments proposed do indeed test the hypothesis. While designing these experiments, it is essential to identify what controls will be needed. Some of these will be controls required for the actual hypothesis testing but in laboratory-based studies there may well be additional controls necessary to ensure that the assay or reagents are working as expected. Specific examples of such studies are given later in this chapter.

Modern biomedical research has developed rapidly in the last 25 years and continues to do so at an increasing pace. The use of cellular and molecular techniques to understand the biochemical and genetic basis of health and disease has radically altered our understanding of physiology. However, to perform such experiments, complex biochemical and/or genetic techniques are required that use many specialised reagents. It is, therefore, of fundamental importance that the reagents, be they antibodies, probes or oligonucleotides, are well characterised and their performance verified during the course of an experimental procedure.

Are you sure you are measuring what you think you are measuring?

In this context, it is of paramount importance that all probes and antibodies are validated for the use to which they are to be put. DNA probes (including oligonucleotides) should be sequenced and checked for specificity. This is particularly important for DNA probes that may contain repeated sequences or are derived from regions of genes which may be conserved. The latter can include control regions of promoters but also functional domains of coding sequences. Derivation of a shorter DNA probe may well actually improve specificity although it can reduce sensitivity.

Validation of antibody performance is more problematic than that for DNA probes and this is particularly true when antibodies are to be used for immuno-histochemistry. Ideally, the performance of an antibody used for immunolocali-sation should be compared with localisation studies using alternative techniques, such as radioligand binding or *in situ* hybridisation. However, this is frequently impossible and therefore you may resort to Western blotting to demonstrate that the antibody indeed recognises an antigen of the expected molecular weight.

While a successful Western blot gives considerable reassurance of the specificity of an antibody, failure to achieve success using this particular technique does not necessarily mean that immunostaining in tissue sections is invalid. For example, if the immunolocalisation is confined to a very rare population of cells in the section, the antigen may be undetectable when tissue is homogenised and analysed by Western blotting. In any event, the appropriate controls must be performed when carrying out immunohistology. These include, for monoclonal antibodies, use of an isotope-matched control and for polyclonal antibodies the use of non-immune serum of the same species (if possible preimmune serum from the same animal). Where the antibody has been raised against a synthetic peptide, preabsorption of the antisera with an excess of the peptide should be performed. However, it is possible still to have spurious staining which appears to be specific, since it can be obliterated by such preabsorption. This is thought to occur because of shared but unidentified epitopes in the peptide, which are also common to several antigens present within the tissue. When describing the results of immunohistochemistry, the experimenter should take care in the description of the result. Specifically, 'antigen-like immunoreactivity' is what has been localised, not the protein, and neither of these equates in any way to a demonstration of gene expression.

Antibodies are also commonly used in radio immunoassays (RIA) and enzyme-linked immunosorbent assays (ELISA); again, using these quantitative assays it is essential that the antibody and antigen labelling are both validated. Antibody specificity is of paramount importance when measuring levels of closely related analytes (for example, related steroid hormones or prostanoids). When such relatively small organic compounds are being assayed, the radiolabel is usually incorporated directly into the antigen and does not alter its chemical structure. However, it is common when measuring peptides, polypeptides and proteins for the radiolabel (or indeed other label) to be chemically attached to the antigen. In such cases, it is essential to demonstrate that the iodination or biotinylation (for example) of the peptide or protein has not resulted in an alteration in antigen immunoreactivity. In addition, it is essential to demonstrate that dilutions of the sample are parallel to dilutions of the standard curve and that 'spike and recover' experiments give reproducible and consistent recoveries. Finally, it is important that internal controls should be included in every assay to allow continuing determination of the inter- and intra-assay coefficients of variation.

These points are clearly of great importance to anyone wishing to develop an immunoassay; however, users of commercial assays should be aware that even these assays need to be validated and, while the purchaser may expect that the supplier of the assay will have carried out such validation, the demonstration of parallelism between the specific samples being used by the researcher and the standard curve is a valuable test to run.

The two examples of Northern blotting and the polymerase chain reaction given below illustrate the steps that need to be taken to ensure that a valid experiment is performed using these techniques. Without validation of the assays, hypothesis testing becomes impossible.

Example 1: Northern blotting

Northern blotting is a widely used and straightforward technique which identifies and possibly quantifies the messenger RNA (mRNA) encoding a specific gene product within a population of RNA isolated from either cells or tissue. However, the apparent simplicity belies the underlying factors every researcher must consider. The points to be considered are:

- Sample selection: this will depend on the hypothesis to be tested but should include appropriate controls, for example treated versus untreated cells or tissues; RNA from affected or unaffected individuals (attention needs to be paid as to how these are identified, how rigorous this selection is and how many replicates of each sample are to be analysed).
- The RNA samples to be run on the gel should all be prepared in the same way, the amount of RNA should be quantified and its integrity demonstrated.
- Appropriate molecular weight markers need to be run on the gel, as do additional samples which demonstrate the specificity of the probe to be used subsequently (a positive and a negative control).
- The gel needs to be run and the RNA transferred to the blotting membrane. Since the RNA can be degraded during each of these processes, some sort of staining of the membrane should be performed on the membrane to demonstrate that RNA has successfully been transferred and is still intact.
- The probe that is to be used in the hybridisation study should be characterised (by DNA sequencing). The purity and concentration of the probe need to be determined prior to labelling and the efficiency of labelling also needs to be determined.
- The hybridisation and washing conditions to be used may need to be refined by preliminary experimentation. However, this is only possible once a suitable positive control and probe have been identified.

- After autoradiography, the probe should be removed and the filter re-probed with an additional probe that hybridises to a housekeeping gene. This serves as a control to demonstrate that the loading of the gel and transfer to the membrane was even and that there was hybridisable RNA present in every lane.

While Northern blotting is one of the simplest techniques used in modern molecular biology, from this list it is obvious that there are numerous steps which can go wrong and which need to be validated during the course of the experiment. While most of them are relatively simple, they should not be overlooked.

Example 2: polymerase chain reaction

The polymerase chain reaction (PCR) is the workhorse of modern molecular biology and is based on the *in vitro* amplification of double-stranded DNA using a thermostable DNA polymerase. Again, its simplicity belies the under-lying complexity and the pitfalls that await the unwary. The key questions to be considered by the researcher in performing these PCR reactions can be summed up in two questions:
- Did the reaction work?
- Was there PCR template present?

Thus, when carrying out such reactions, it is essential to include controls to demonstrate that the primers, enzyme and buffer are all functioning and that the template added (cDNA or genomic DNA) can be successfully amplified using alternative primers. An additional control that is absolutely essential for PCR reactions is the 'no-template control'. This demonstrates that there was no contamination of any of the reagents with a small amount of template, which would lead to a false positive result. The importance of this negative control cannot be emphasised enough since, owing to the extreme sensitivity of the PCR reaction, very small amounts of contamination can easily lead to false positive results.

An example where all these considerations have been taken into account is shown in Figure 11.1. From this example, it can be seen that all the controls described above are included. This specific experiment set out to determine whether acidic fibroblast growth factor (FGF) and basic FGF were expressed in the two endometrial carcinoma cell lines HEC1-A and HEC1-B. Thus, the integrity of the RNA and the PCR ability of the cDNA was tested by ampli-fying cDNA from these two cell lines and also from normal proliferative phase endometrium with primers specifically for vascular endothelial growth factor (VEGF). These samples are shown in lanes 2, 3 and 4. Lane 5 contains a negative control with no template, showing that the VEGF PCR reaction was not contaminated. Lanes 6 and 7 demonstrate that the PCR reaction designed to amplify acidic and basic FGF cDNA also worked when using

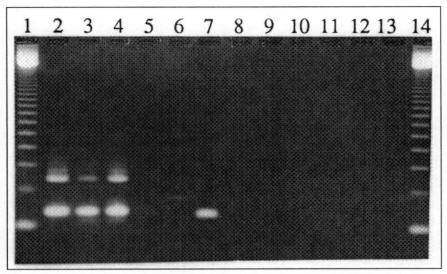

Figure 11.1 Agarose gel showing PCR products from the amplification of cDNA from the proliferative endometrium (lanes 2, 6 and 7), HEC1-A (lanes 3, 8 and 9), HEC1-B cell line (lanes 4, 10 and 11) and control (no template) (lanes 5, 12 and 13), with nested primers specific to VEGF (lanes 2, 3, 4 and 5), acidic FGF (lanes 6, 8, 10 and 12) and basic FGF (lanes 7, 9, 11 and 13). Lanes 1 and 14 are molecular weight markers (123bp ladder, BRL). Reproduced from Charnock-Jones et al. (1993) with permission[1]

cDNA from proliferative phase endometrium. The negative controls demonstrating absence of contamination for the acidic and basic FGF PCR reactions are in lanes 12 and 13. The actual experimental lanes are lanes 8, 9, 10 and 11, in which cDNA from the two cell lines is amplified with primers specific for acidic or basic FGF. As can be seen, no PCR product is produced by these reactions. However, the other lanes on the gel demonstrate that the PCR reactions for acidic and basic FGF worked and that there was indeed intact cDNA present in the samples derived from the two cell lines in question. Thus, one can reliably conclude that acidic and basic FGF mRNA were either absent or below the level of sensitivity in this assay in the two endometrial carcinoma cell lines HEC1-A and HEC1-B.

Having formulated the hypothesis, designed rational experiments and carried them out using all the controls necessary both to validate the assays used and also as required by the hypothesis, you are left with the interpretation. A temptation at this point is to over-interpret the data and this should be resisted. For example, a common failing is to suggest that immunohistochemical localisation of an antigen means that there is local expression of the protein of interest. This is not the case. Strictly speaking, immunohistochemical localisation shows that there is an antigen-like immunoreactivity.

Conclusion

The essentials for good-quality laboratory research can be summed up as follows:

- Have a good clear simple hypothesis.
- Design relevant experiments, which test this.
- Perform experiments as designed, with the appropriate controls as required for the hypothesis and assay validation.
- Interpret cautiously.

Reference

1. Charnock-Jones, DS, Sharkey, AM, Rajput-Williams J, Burch D, Schofield JP, Fountain SA, *et al*. Identification and localization of alternately spliced mRNAs for vascular endothelial growth factor in human uterus and estrogen regulation in endometrial carcinoma cell lines. *Biol Reprod* 1993;48:1120–8.

12

Data management

Kirstie McKenzie-McHarg and Sarah Ayers

Introduction

Data management is a broad issue and this chapter details the themes that must be considered when you are planning and undertaking your research project. Once the research question has been formulated, the appropriate study design selected, the protocol written and funding and ethics approval obtained, answering your research question accurately depends entirely on the data. Regardless of the size or methodology of the project, obtaining a complete and accurate data set should be your highest priority. Without valid, accurate, accessible and verifiable data you cannot obtain a reliable result. Therefore, putting efficient data management systems into place early is crucial. Good data management is simple but requires a little thought, preferably before data collection begins.

Data management systems will necessarily vary immensely depending on your research design. You may be conducting a laboratory-based study, with all data being collected, collated and analysed by one person. At the more complex end, you may be running a large, multicentre study, involving hundreds of centres and thousands of subjects. In this chapter, we have assumed the most complex situation and will leave it to you to extract the information that best fits your needs.

What are the data?

The data comprise every single item of information you collect for your study. Unfortunately, it is all too easy to design a study, collect the data and then discover that you have not recorded the information in a way that will allow you to answer the research question in which you are interested. Therefore, it is crucial that you think about your final questions and what data you will need to answer these questions. It is also important that you do not collect redundant data: data that you will not use to answer the research questions in which you have an interest. Collecting redundant data wastes your time and the time of any others involved in collecting them. In multicentre trials, there are sometimes 'dummy tables' to help you decide what data to collect. These should comprise the final data tables (blank, of course) which, as far as possible, will be used to produce the study results as defined in the protocol. However, for all studies, it is certainly worth spending some time considering the data you will need to collect to answer your research questions carefully and the forms that you will use to record the data you collect. Even in the case of a small, laboratory-based study, it is always worth producing a form for data collection. This ensures that your procedure is standardised and items are not missed. It makes checking your data easier and provides a record that will exist after the study is completed.

It is a good idea to ask people unconnected with the project to look at the forms or to try completing them to look for ambiguities and other problems that may not be apparent to the person designing the form. If at all possible, the forms should be piloted among the people who are going to be completing them in the final study. For example, if you are interested in recruiting women at 24–30 weeks of gestation, pilot your forms among a sample of pregnant women of that gestation. Women earlier or later in their pregnancy could be in a different situation, which may mean that the pilot does not pick up common problems. Once you have tested and verified the data form, the project can begin.

The issues involved in managing the data, once they are gathered, are numerous and each requires some preparation:

- complying with the 1998 Data Protection Act
- dealing with data on a day-to-day basis
- following up missing data coding
- distinguishing missing data from data indicated as unknown (this is an important question which is often ignored)
- staff
- preparing for analysis
- deciding whether your data will be collected electronically or in paper format
- deciding how your data will be stored and backed up.

The 1998 Data Protection Act

The 1998 Data Protection Act states that every effort must be made to maintain confidentiality of personal data held on computer or stored in locked filing cabinets. Simultaneously, the system you devise needs to be workable, allowing authorised people easy access to data when needed, while preventing unauthorised access. This implies that all paperwork containing confidential or identifiable information should be locked away at all times, with restricted access to it, as well as restricted access to any data held on computer. The Act also suggests that names and addresses should be stored separately from main outcome data so that non-project staff cannot link them together. This applies to both electronic and paper data. The requirements of the 1998 Data Protection Act vary, depending on the type of study you are undertaking and the type of data being collected, and it is not possible for us to generalise. However, it should be stressed that you must comply with the requirement of the Act and you should ensure that you fully understand the requirements of the Act with regard to your study. Further information about the 1998 Data

Protection Act can be obtained from www.informationcommissioner.gov. uk.

Managing data on a day-to-day basis

This is where the type of research study you are conducting could have an enormous impact on the work you need to do in order to deal with your data efficiently. Again, we have assumed the most complex situation and a number of these points will not apply if you are collecting all the data yourself. However, many of the points are true regardless of the size of your project.

One of the first things you need to do is to develop a procedure for managing the data forms when they begin returning to the study office. We rec-

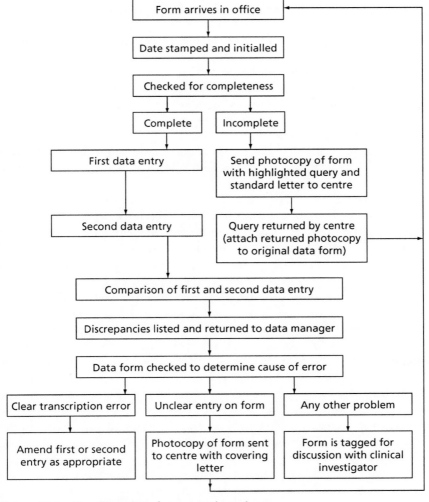

Figure 12.1 Handling data for research projects

ommend that you make this procedure a high priority on your list of tasks. You might want to consider something along the following lines (Figure 12.1).

- Data forms should be date-stamped on arrival, checked for completeness and 'checked in' – in other words, the arrival of the form is recorded, either electronically or on paper.

- If omissions or incomplete forms are discovered at this first check, you need to decide if it will be possible to obtain the missing data; for example, a date of birth should always be available; a specific item on a profession-ally administered questionnaire which was omitted at the time will not be available and will be coded as permanently missing. If you decide to try to obtain the missing data then you should return a photocopy of the data form, highlighting the omission or error to the study centre together with a covering letter. The original data form should never be returned to the person who completed it asking them to resolve a query (you might never see it again).

- Once a form is complete, it should be filed in a manner that means you can find it again easily; most studies allocate a unique number to each subject and file paperwork consecutively by these subject numbers.

Following up missing data

In the search for a complete and accurate data set, the following up of missing data is one of the most crucial elements. This could take one of several forms.

In the first case, you may be awaiting data from an individual or an organ-isation (such as a hospital ward, GP clinic or NHS trust) that has not yet returned a questionnaire or data collection form. In the first instance, a system of automatic reminders should be instigated. The specifics of your project will play some part in helping you to decide how many postal reminders will be appropriate before you begin telephoning. If you are collecting informa-tion from a mother whose baby has died recently, it is unlikely that you would wish to contact her too often; however, if it is a case of determining a patient's blood pressure at a given moment from hospital case notes, you may need to contact the hospital frequently to obtain the information you need. In some situations, it may be necessary to visit the hospital yourself to obtain the information you need but, as this obviously adds cost to your project, it is to be avoided; instead, concentrate on vigorous and frequent reminders regard-ing your missing form. If it does become imperative that you visit the hospi-tal, you might require an honorary contract in order to gain access to the medical notes. This is obviously time consuming and complex and may not be possible within some trusts.

A second case could be where a questionnaire or form has been returned to you but is incomplete in some detail. As you should not be collecting unimportant information, you should make every effort to pursue the missing data. As stated earlier, you should never send a form out of the data office once received. Instead, you should copy the original and send the copy, with missing information highlighted, to the person responsible for completing the form, together with a letter asking them to supply the missing information. A flowchart of this process is included in Figure 12.1. Again, a series of reminders should be instigated so that organisations are contacted on a regular basis until the missing piece of information is either found or you are told categorically that it is unavailable.

Coding

Once you have all the data that you can possibly obtain in your possession, coding may need to take place. Some forms of qualitative research (see Chapter 13 for a description of qualitative and quantitative research), especially those demanding content analysis, may require the transcription of conversations or written answers word for word and specialised software packages are available to assist in this type of work. Do consider using one of these packages if it is warranted, as it can assist you in the analysis of your project.

Quantitative research, however, is unlikely to require lengthy text answers and most data can be coded for ease of analysis. By coding, we mean that a text response is given a code that makes it easier to handle at the analysis stage. For example, if you are asking about use of analgesia then you might want to use '1' for aspirin, '2' for paracetamol, '3' for codeine, and so on. Using the numeric code instead of the text means that misspellings and other transcription errors become less important. If you are not doing this yourself but using data entry clerks, it is important to ensure that data are double-entered (see 'Preparing for analysis' below) and that you are available to check forms which have queries. In some cases, the individual completing the form may need to be contacted to clarify their response to your question.

Distinguishing missing data from data that are unknown

It is at this time that a distinction should be made between data indicated as 'unknown' by the person completing the form (the piece of information you are requesting was never collected and hence is not known) and data which are 'missing' (information you have requested does exist but the person completing the form either cannot or will not find it). This allows you to make a judgement about the benefit of including a question that may have (for example) a 65% response rate of 'unknown' but a 'missing' response rate of only 5%. Similarly, if a question requires the person answering it to find information elsewhere, you may have a very high 'missing' rate and the question therefore may be deemed unsuitable. It is useful to code your missing data so that you can categorise it. The most usual way to do this is to use different codes, such as:

- '9' (or '99' or '999' depending on your specific data item) for 'not known and will remain not known'

- '8' for 'not applicable in this case'
- '7' for 'not known but we are chasing this data item'.

This is the benefit of pilot studies, which allow you to determine all this before commencing a large project. If during the pilot study you find that a crucial question in terms of your research is either frequently unknown or often missing, you may need to think of alternative methods of addressing your question.

Data collection: electronic or paper format?

How do you decide if your data should be collected and analysed on paper or electronically? There are clear benefits and disadvantages in each case. In the case of electronic data collection, the data are entered immediately, at source, into a computer and the data saved on disk. This is quick and has the benefit of requiring little physical storage space. However, it can be difficult to decide how to handle unexpected responses when you are sitting in front of the computer and the respondent is waiting for you to move on to the next question. In addition, information entered directly into a computer cannot be verified and usually cannot be double-entered, unless this is done twice at the point of origin.

In the case of data collection on paper, there is a clear disadvantage in terms of physical storage space required. However, there are many benefits of paper data collection. The first is that you have a permanent paper record of the answer to a question, to which any queries may be referred. In addition, data entry can be conducted at convenient times and if the answer to a question appears incorrect, this can be checked by returning a copy to the person responsible for completing it. On balance, paper data collection (with subsequent entry on to computer if appropriate) tends to be more accurate.

Staff

The number of staff you employ to conduct a project will depend entirely on the amount of data being collected. If the project is relatively small and has very little money, it may be that you will do everything yourself. In this case, every effort should be made to find somebody else willing to do second data entry for you so that the accuracy of your data set will not be challenged. At the other extreme are very large randomised controlled trials. Some of these trials may require you to collect data from thousands of subjects and you will need staff to run the project efficiently.

There are several options you can consider in terms of staff for a large project. In the case of electronic data being collected at source, at least two people will need to be identified in each centre collecting data, in order to do double data entry and a computer programmer may be needed to set up the initial systems and prepare data for analysis. No further staff are necessary; any missing data in this system remain missing forever, as there are no paper copies to return to respondents with requests for further information. In the case of paper data collection, you could consider employing a data manager, whose job it is to ensure that the data set is as complete and accurate as possible and who is in charge of following up all missing data. If you wish, the data manager could also be responsible for first data entry – this will depend on the size of the project. A second person to conduct second data entry will also be required, as well as a computer programmer. If the project is very large, two data entry clerks may be needed in addition to the data manager in order to complete the data entry.

Preparing for analysis

You should consider how to handle analysis of your data. Should this be on paper (only for a small project) or have you entered the data on to a custom-designed computer database, spreadsheet or other software package? For a large project, you might also consider specialised scanning software, which would enable you to scan your data forms. This has become a more realistic option with improvements in electronic technology.

If you have entered the data on to a computer then, as stated previously, we would strongly recommend using double data entry to minimise typing errors, difficulties of interpretation of illegible handwriting, and so on. The two sets of data should have been entered by two different people on two separate occasions without conferring. If there are discrepancies between first and second data entry, there are two options. If you have a customised data entry program then, at the time of second entry, an error message could appear on the screen if a discrepancy is noted by the computer program. This message informs the second data entry person that the value just entered is different from the value entered by the first person. The second data entry person can then check the paper copy and make a decision as to the correct answer. The disadvantage of this system is that the person doing second data entry is unlikely to be qualified to make such decisions. For example, if it is a clinical question, then it should be referred to the appropriate person. Therefore, a second option is that a printout of discrepancies can be produced after all data entry is completed. Computer software is available which will do this. This list is presented to the appropriate person, who can make decisions based on whether the discrepancy is due to simple error at the time of data entry, an error due to unclear handwriting (which may need to be verified with the person completing the form) or an error due to any other reason.

Any annotations to data forms should be in a different coloured ink, should not obliterate the original entry and must be initialled and dated by the data manager or principal investigator. An additional safeguard is to have an 'audit trail' built into your computer program. Any changes to the data are recorded with the initials of the person making the change and the date, so that changes can be followed through later. This has overheads in terms of computer programming and storage space required but is well worth doing if at all possible, particularly for larger projects.

Storing and backing up data

Finally, perhaps the most crucial element of your research is the backing-up of your data. There are often plaintive advertisements in the newspapers saying 'Lost/stolen, laptop computer containing the only record of x years' work'. Do not put yourself in this position. After spending considerable time and energy obtaining a complete data set, you do not want to lose it to a computer malfunction or theft. All data should be backed up on a regular basis – certainly not less than weekly and preferably daily – and the backup stored in a separate location. You can back up your data manually on to memory stick, CD-ROM or DVD or purchase back up software in the case of a larger study. You should remove at least one copy of the data from the building in which the original data set is held and update this copy regularly. In addition, you must make sure that you can restore your data from the backup disks. All too often, the crucial backups are found to be unusable at the very time they are needed.

Conclusion

In conclusion, the systems used to ensure good data management are not complex but they are important. Thinking about these systems at the outset of your project will save you a great deal of time and energy and should ensure that you gather the best possible data, resulting in a far better research project. Good luck!

13

Statistics

Peter Brocklehurst and Simon Gates

Introduction

In this chapter we aim to give a basic introduction to the main concepts involved in planning and undertaking statistical analysis and to indicate what methods of analysis should be used in common situations. We do not give details of how to carry out the statistical tests. These can be found in many statistics textbooks and a list of suitable reference books is provided at the end of the chapter. The examples used to illustrate some of the statistical concepts are predominantly clinical studies, but the concepts apply equally to other research settings, such as laboratory-based studies.

Why we need statistics

Statistics are necessary because of the intrinsic variability of humans and animals. Every individual who could be included in a research study is different and will respond differently to an intervention or exposure to a risk factor. A group of subjects who experience the same intervention or risk factor will, therefore, not all respond in the same way but there will be a range of responses. In a research study, we usually want to discover whether there is a difference between two or more groups of individuals who have been given different treatments or have experienced different exposures. The individuals in each group will differ just by chance, so in each group there will be a range of responses. To find out whether the different treatments have any effect on the outcome we need to separate the effects of chance variation from those of the treatment. Statistical methods provide ways of doing this: they help us to understand the relationships between variables and to draw valid conclusions.

What statistical methods are used for

Statistical methods are used for three purposes:

- Summarising data for presentation, by means of summary statistics and graphs. Summary statistics measure the central characteristic of a set of data and the spread around it, for example by the mean and standard deviation or the median and interquartile range.
- Finding out how likely it is that the data obtained in a study could have arisen by chance and, hence, how likely it is that there is a real difference between the groups studied.

- Assessing the reliability of results and generalising from the individuals in the study to the whole population of which they are part. For example, if a study is carried out in 100 pregnant women, the result will depend partly on the characteristics of these women and would be slightly different if a different set of 100 women were selected. Statistical methods enable us to assess how well the result from the individuals in the study represents the whole of the population from which they are drawn.

Planning statistical analyses

The key to easy and successful analysis is planning. Before data collection is started, it is essential to know:

- what data will be collected and what will then be done with them
- what comparisons will be made and what statistical procedures will be used.

Without adequate planning, you run the risk of failing to collect all of the necessary data or of wasting effort on gathering data that are impossible to analyse. Collecting data is difficult and expensive, so it pays to be clear at the outset exactly what data will be collected and what will not. Writing a study protocol is essential. This should contain as much detail as possible on:

- what data will be collected
- the methods of data collection
- sample size calculations (see Chapter 8)
- methods of analysis.

The analysis is an important part of the project, so it should be included in the plan which is drawn up at the start. You should discuss the study while you are planning it with researchers and statisticians who have experience in the type of study design and analytical methods that you propose to use. At this stage, you can make changes to your plans in the light of other people's experience and expertise.

Types of data

The type of analysis that is performed will depend on what questions are to be asked and on the types of data that have been collected. Different sorts of data require different sorts of analysis and you should be careful not to use statistical tests that are inappropriate for your data, as doing so may give erroneous results.

Continuous variables are those that are measured on a continuous scale, such as height and weight. Discrete variables can take only certain values, such as the number of cases of a disease in a week, which can only be a whole number. Categorical variables are ones where each individual is in one of a number of mutually exclusive classes, such as country of birth, sex or type of drug. Categorical variables may be ordered, where the categories form a natural sequence. For example, the number of children a woman has is an ordered categorical, whereas country of birth is not ordered. Binary variables are an important type of categorical variable, where there are only two classes such as yes or no, alive or dead, preterm or term.

For many variables, if a plot is made of each value against its frequency in a large number of people, the resulting graph will have a characteristic symmetrical bell shape. Birth weight is an example of such a variable; the most common value is the mean birth weight and the majority of people have a birth weight fairly close to this. Extremely high or low birth weights are much rarer. A plot such as this of the frequency of occurrence of each possible value shows the distribution of the data and the symmetrical bell-shaped curve is known as a normal distribution. There are many possible distributions of data; some examples are shown in Figure 13.1.

The distribution of the data is important because it affects the way the analysis is performed. Some statistical methods require that the data are sampled from a normal distribution (see 'Parametric statistics', below) and, if this is not the case, other methods should be used.

It can sometimes be more meaningful to present continuous data as categorical variables. For example, suppose that, in a randomised controlled trial (RCT) comparing two operative techniques, the mean blood loss was 435 ml in the group given the new treatment and 389 ml in the conventional treatment group. If the question of interest is whether the patients had any major blood loss, these figures are uninformative. An alternative way of presenting the same data would be to calculate the proportion of patients in each group who lost more than 500 ml at operation: 41% in the new treatment group and 38% in the conventional treatment group. How to present data depends on what information the investigators wish to convey and a continuous outcome sometimes fails to convey the relevant information.

The outcome being measured is often referred to as the response variable, to distinguish it from the explanatory variable or variables. For example, in an experiment comparing two drug treatments for hypertension in pregnancy, the response variable would be blood pressure and the explanatory variable would be a categorical variable with two classes, one for each drug.

Risks and odds

Binary response variables, where each individual has one of two possible outcomes, are usually presented as risks or odds. These are ways of summarising the data and making comparisons between groups. The risk is the proportion of the group under study who develop the outcome of interest. For instance, if 1000 primigravid women are followed throughout their pregnancy and 20 of them develop gestational diabetes, the risk of developing gestational diabetes in this group is 20/1000 or 2%.

The odds is the ratio of the number of a group who develop the outcome of interest to the number who do not. Using the example above, the odds of

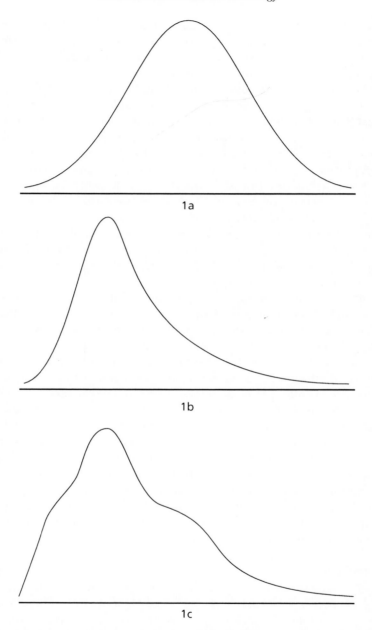

Figure 13.1   Some examples of distributions of variables: (a) a normal distribution; (b) a non-normal distribution; this one is asymmetrical, with a 'tail' on the right; (c) a different non-normal distribution; this one has a complex shape

developing gestational diabetes are 20/(1000 – 20) = 20/980 = 2.04%. As this example demonstrates, when the outcome is uncommon, the odds are very similar to the risk. Odds rather than risks have to be used where the total population at risk is not known, so a risk cannot be calculated; for example, in case–control studies (see Chapter 14).

The most common use for odds or risks is in comparisons of two groups; a ratio of the odds (the odds ratio, OR) or risk (relative risk, RR) between the two groups is calculated and this gives a measure of the difference between the groups. Confidence intervals can be calculated for the OR or RR and results are commonly presented in this way (see 'Comparing proportions', below).

As an example of the calculation of the OR and RR, consider an RCT investigating the effects of two different antibiotic regimens for the prevention of postoperative infection. A table can be constructed (Table 13.1). From this, the OR and the RR can be calculated:

$$\text{Odds ratio} = \frac{\text{Odds of infection with antibiotic A}}{\text{Odds of infection with antibiotic B}}$$

$$= \frac{(\text{Infections with antibiotic A/No infections with antibiotic A})}{(\text{Infections with antibiotic B/No infections with antibiotic B})}$$

$$= \frac{23/85}{40/66}$$

$$= 0.45$$

$$\text{Relative risk} = \frac{\text{Risk of infection with A}}{\text{Risk of infection with B}}$$

$$= \frac{(\text{Number infected with antibiotic A/Total number given antibiotic A})}{(\text{Number infected with antibiotic B/Total number given antibiotic B})}$$

$$= \frac{23/(85+23)}{40/(66+40)}$$

$$= 0.56$$

The interpretation of these results is that antibiotic A is associated with a halving of the incidence of postoperative infection compared with antibiotic B.

Table 13.1 A table to calculate the odds ratio and relative risk		
	Infections	No infections
Antibiotic A	23	85
Antibiotic B	40	66

Concepts involved in statistical analysis

Confidence intervals

Because the individuals included in a research study are a sample from a larger population, it is important to know how well the study's results reflect the true value for the whole population. For example, a study might be carried out on 100 pregnant women. How well does the result for these women match the result that would be obtained if all pregnant women could be studied? Confidence intervals provide a way of measuring the reliability of results, by giving a range around the result within which you would reasonably expect the true value for the population to lie. If the confidence interval is wide, there is a wide range of values which the true value could be, so the result is a poor estimate of it. If the confidence interval is narrow, the result measures the true value in the population fairly precisely. Usually, 95% confidence intervals are calculated, which give a range that will include the true value with a probability of 0.95.

Hypothesis testing

Hypothesis testing is the process by which we can ask how likely it is that an observed result is due to chance alone. To do this, a wide variety of statistical tests exists, which all work in the same basic way: they work out how likely it is that the observed data would have been obtained if there were really no difference between the groups. The hypothesis that there is no difference is known as the null hypothesis. Statistical tests express this likelihood as a probability, known as the P value. A high P value means that you can accept the null hypothesis and conclude that there is no difference between your groups. If the P value is low, you can reject the null hypothesis and conclude that there is a real difference. The convention has arisen of using a P value of 0.05 as the cut-off for whether two groups are considered 'significantly' different. This means that the existence of a real difference is concluded if the probability is less than 0.05, or in other words, if there is less than a 1 in 20 chance that the result is due simply to random variation.

The main problem with P values is that they tell you nothing about the size of the difference between the groups. If the sample size is very large, a P value of less than 0.05 can result from a very small and clinically unimportant difference. Conversely, if the sample size is small, a large and potentially clinically important difference may yield a P value of greater than 0.05. For this reason, it is not recommended to present results simply as P values. It is much more informative to present an estimate of the size of the difference between groups together with a confidence interval.

Power

Statistical tests are not completely reliable and there is a chance that a test will fail to discover a real difference, even though there is one. The probability that a test will discover a real difference is called its power. Power is influenced by sample size and by the size of the difference – a larger difference will be easier to detect and will give the test more power, as will a larger sample size. Failure to find a difference between two groups may be because none exists or it may be because of lack of power in the test. It is important to consider statistical power in planning what sample size is necessary in your study; the study must be large enough to give the test used sufficient power to provide an answer to the question being investigated.

Parametric and non-parametric statistics

Statistical tests can be broadly divided into parametric and non-parametric tests. The essential difference between them is that parametric statistics make assumptions about the distribution of the data, as they involve calculating parameters from the data, whereas non-parametric statistics do not (hence their alternative name 'distribution-free statistics'). If you use parametric statistics, it is important that their assumptions are met; if not, or if there is doubt about this, non-parametric statistics should be preferred. One of the most common assumptions of parametric statistics is that the data should be normally distributed. Many common measurements, such as length of post-surgical hospital stay, operating time and duration of labour, are not normally distributed; their distributions are asymmetrical because there are a few people for which these durations are very long. In these cases, either non-parametric methods should be used or the data should be transformed. Transformation simply means subjecting all of the values of the response variable to some mathematical operation, such as taking logarithms, so that the data become normally distributed. If the transformation is successful, they can then be analysed using parametric methods. Alternatively, continuous data can be changed to a categorical variable (for example, the length of stay in hospital after hysterectomy could be changed to the number of women in hospital for more than 7 days after their operation) and the groups can then be compared using parametric methods.

Carrying out statistical analyses

Exploratory analysis

The first step in an analysis should be to familiarise yourself with the data, by calculating summary statistics, creating tables and plotting graphs. If you are comparing a normally distributed continuous variable between two groups, the mean and standard deviation (SD) for each group should be calculated. With a non-normally distributed continuous variable, the median value represents the central characteristic of the data and the interquartile range represents its spread. If you are looking for an association between two continuous variables, plot the two variables against each other. If your response variable is categorical, tables of counts and proportions are appropriate.

These exploratory steps will help you to see any features of the data that were not anticipated that you may need to explore further in your analysis. For example, you may have anticipated a linear relationship between two continuous variables. However, a graph of the data may suggest that it is actually curved. This can then be incorporated into the analysis; you can carry out a test to see if a curve fits the data better than a straight line. Furthermore, this sort of examination of the data can highlight any errors in the data and reveal any data points that look very different from the rest (known as 'outliers'). These should be investigated carefully: has something atypical happened to those individuals or have the data not been recorded correctly?

Statistical software

Virtually all analyses are done by computer and many large and comprehensive software packages (such as SAS, SPSS, Stata and Minitab) are available. These can give you all of the statistics you are likely to need. Which to use is largely a matter of personal preference. There are two common problems with statistical software:

- They will often produce answers uncritically, even if the analysis you are running is inappropriate. The computer can do complicated calculations easily but the analyst still needs to know what he or she is doing.
- Their output can be confusing, sometimes producing pages of output from a simple test. Manuals supplied with the software may be unhelpful, so it is advisable to refer to someone who is experienced with the software you propose to use.

Methods of analysis

Comparing means

When a study compares two groups in which the outcome is a continuous variable, the means of the two groups can be compared. For example, in a study comparing birth weight in two groups of babies, the mean of the first group of 206 babies is 3254 g (SD 438 g) and that of the other group of 184 babies is 3602 g (SD 509 g). There are several ways of comparing these data and the method used will depend on what information the investigators wish to convey. If the purpose is to demonstrate that the difference between the two groups is unlikely to have occurred by chance, then a Student's t-test will produce a P value (for this example, the P value is less than 0.001, so this difference in birth weight is unlikely to have occurred by chance). However, to determine not only whether a difference exists but also to find out how large it is, then the difference in mean birth weight can be calculated, together with a confidence interval, which expresses the uncertainty around the estimate of the difference. In this example, the difference between the means is 348 g, 95% confidence interval 254–442 g. Therefore, the difference between the birth weights of these two groups of women is between 254 g and 442 g. This

— 156 —

is unlikely to have occurred by chance, as the range does not include 0 or a negative value.

Another way to compare these data would be to compare the incidence of low birth weight (less than 2500 g) in each group; that is, convert birth weight into a categorical variable.

The non-parametric equivalent of the Student's t-test is the Mann–Whitney test.

Comparing more than two means

If there are more than two groups to be compared, the approach used will depend on what information the investigators wish to convey. If there are four groups of women and each group has a mean postoperative haemoglobin, then comparing each of three groups with one 'baseline' group (which would usually be the control treatment) may be the approach which is adopted. This will yield three P values or three mean differences, each with a 95% confidence interval (as above). Alternatively, the investigators may simply want to investigate whether the four groups are different from each other, in which case an analysis of variance (ANOVA) can be performed and a P value will result. If a non-parametric test is needed, the Mann–Whitney tests can be used for pair-wise comparisons, and the Kruskal–Wallis test is the equivalent of the ANOVA.

Comparing proportions

If the outcome is measured as a binary variable, the proportion of individuals who have it in each group can be compared. As with comparing means, various methods can be used depending on the question being addressed. If the aim is to determine whether the two proportions are different and whether this difference is unlikely to be due to chance then a chi-square test is appropriate and will yield a P value. However, if the aim is to estimate how different two proportions are then the difference between them and a 95% confidence interval for this difference can be presented. Alternatively, the OR or RR between the two groups with its 95% confidence interval can be calculated. For example, an RCT which aims to determine the proportion of women who continue to experience climacteric symptoms with a new treatment finds that 20% (124/620) of women in the standard treatment group have persistent symptoms compared with 11% (66/598) in the new treatment group. Is this different?

A chi-square test produces a P value of < 0.001, suggesting that the difference is unlikely to be due to chance. The difference in proportions is 9%, with a 95% confidence interval of 5–13%, suggesting that 5–13% fewer women in the new treatment group have persistent symptoms. The OR is 0.50, with a 95% confidence interval of 0.35–0.69, suggesting that women in the new treatment group are between 35% and 69% less likely to have persistent symptoms than those in the standard treatment group.

When comparing proportions between the groups of an ordered categorical variable, for example birthweight groups, a test-for-trend can be performed (in some software packages, this is found under analysis of variance). This will produce a *P* value and will demonstrate whether the distribution of birth weights within the two groups of women is different. The advantage of comparing groups using a test-for-trend is an increase in the power of the test to detect more modest differences than a simple comparison of two groups (for example, < 2500 g and ≥ 2500 g).

Association between continuous variables
If both the explanatory and response variable are continuous, they can be analysed by correlation (Figure 13.2) or linear regression (Figure 13.3). Which of these to use depends on the question being asked. Regression supposes that the response variable depends on the explanatory variable and produces an equation relating them and a *P* value. Correlation does not assume that one variable causes the other, but simply measures their association, by means of a correlation coefficient. This can be between –1 and +1, with 0 representing no association, –1 perfect negative association and +1 perfect positive association. Perfect correlation does not always mean perfect agreement. Consider a comparison of two methods for measuring neonatal bilirubin. There may be perfect correlation but one test may always produce a lower reading than the other. There are both parametric and non-parametric correlation coefficients. The non-parametric version uses a ranking of the data rather than the actual values. To test such a comparison between two tests, the Bland–Altman test of agreement may be more appropriate.

Confounding
Accounting for confounding (see Chapter 14) in the analysis of a study can be performed using stratification or multiple regression analysis. Stratification, at its simplest, involves setting up two-by-two tables for each level of the confounding variable. For example, when trying to determine whether coffee drinking in pregnancy is associated with preterm delivery the following results table may be constructed (Table 13.2). A potential confounder of this association could be cigarette smoking and the analysis can be stratified by whether the women smoked during their pregnancy or not. In reality, smoking status is usually split into more detailed levels but, for the purposes of illustration, the variable will be divided into 'yes' and 'no'. Another table (Table 13.3) can now be constructed.

The results from the stratified tables can be combined using, for example, the Mantel–Haenszel method. This will produce a summary OR of the association between coffee drinking and preterm delivery which has been 'adjusted' for smoking. Stratified analyses are straightforward to carry out and simple to understand but cannot control for more than a small number of confounders at one time. Where it is necessary to control for several confounders simulta-

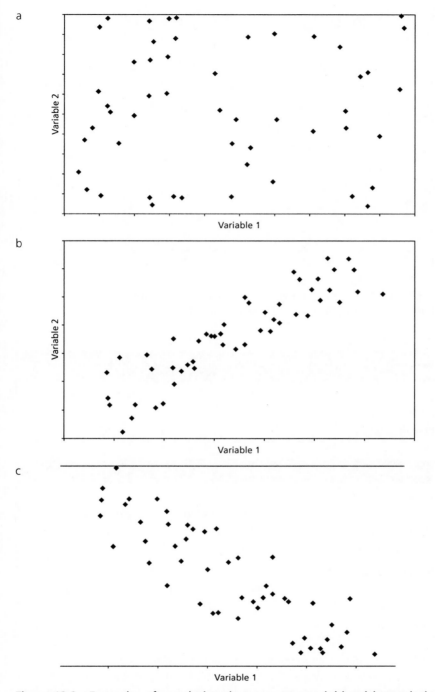

Figure 13.2 Examples of correlations between two variables: (a) correlation coefficient of zero; (b) a positive correlation; (c) a negative correlation

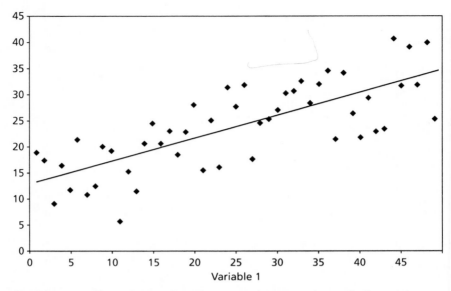

Figure 13.3 A linear regression; the regression procedure calculates a best-fit line through the data, and produces the equation of this line and a *P* value

Table 13.2 The association between coffee drinking and preterm delivery (OR = 1.9)		
	Preterm delivery	**Term delivery**
Coffee drinkers	36	364
Non-coffee drinkers	39	560

Table 13.3 Smokers versus non-smokers		
Smokers (OR = 1.2)		
	Preterm delivery	**Term delivery**
Coffee drinkers	17	120
Non-coffee drinkers	12	97
Non-smokers (OR = 1.3)		
	Preterm delivery	**Term delivery**
Coffee drinkers	19	244
Non-coffee drinkers	27	463

neously, multivariate analyses can be used, of which the most common is multiple regression analysis. The main problem with this technique is that, as the calculations have to be carried out by computer, the data can be simply fed into the 'model' and a result appears without any clear understanding of the data or the modelling process. The properties of the data and the way the model is constructed can affect the results and, for this reason, multiple regression analysis should only be attempted under close supervision by a statistician experienced with this method.

Meta-analysis

The results of individual studies are subject to the same sort of random variation as affects individual subjects within studies. When several studies have addressed the same question, it is desirable that their results should be summarised in some way and the overall result from all of the studies estimated. This should give a more accurate estimate of the true effect than can be gained from any individual study. The statistical methods for combining studies in this way are known as 'meta-analysis'. Several methods exist for carrying out such analyses. In essence, the methods are similar to stratification mentioned above, but the strata (the individual studies) are weighted by some measures, usually the size of the study. It is crucial to the success of meta-analysis that all existing studies are included. Basing the analysis only on well-known studies is likely to introduce bias, as studies showing a large effect may be more likely to be published or widely publicised.

Bayesian analysis

Bayesian analysis is a different approach to statistical analysis. It aims to incorporate into the analysis what was known or believed before the study began and it produces a composite result, combining what has been observed in the study with previous knowledge. Previous knowledge is represented as a probability distribution (the 'prior distribution'), which shows the probability of the possible outcomes. This is modified by the new data to produce a new distribution (the 'posterior distribution'), which represents the probability of the range of outcomes given the information from both sets of data. Bayesian analysis is becoming more widely used but is still controversial.

Further reading

Abelson RP. *Statistics as Principled Argument*. Hillsdale, NJ: Lawrence Erlbaum Associates; 1995.

Altman DG. *Practical Statistics for Medical Research*. London: Chapman and Hall; 1991.

Bland M. *An Introduction to Medical Statistics*. Oxford: Oxford University Press; 1995.

Gardner MJ, Altman D.G. *Statistics With Confidence*. London: BMJ Publishing Group; 1989.

Kirkwood, BR. *Essentials of Medical Statistics*. Oxford: Blackwell Scientific Publications; 1988.

Swinscow TDV. *Statistics at Square One*. 7th ed. London: British Medical Association; 1980.

14

Epidemiology

Paul B Silcocks

What is epidemiology?

Loosely speaking, epidemiology is the study of diseases in defined populations. In some ways it can be thought of as the population equivalent of pathology in the individual but epidemiology is also a branch of applied statistics, motivated by practical medical problems. While numeracy is important, it is not necessary to have a degree in mathematics to contribute to the subject or to derive benefit from an epidemiological approach to medicine.

Branches of epidemiology

Descriptive

Descriptive epidemiology provides general statements on the occurrence of disease by attributes such as age, sex, occupation, class, race, geographic location and calendar period. This information is basic to public health and hypothesis generation. Sources of information include routinely available mortality statistics and cancer registrations and also the results of *ad hoc* surveys.

Analytic

'Analytic' epidemiological studies test ideas relating to the cause, classification, diagnosis or outcome of a disease. Examples are whether smoking causes cervical cancer, how the performance of cytological screening can be evaluated and what factors influence survival. The randomised controlled trial (RCT) can be thought of as a very specialised but highly developed instance of analytic epidemiology.

Theoretical

Theoretical epidemiology is based on mathematical models to simulate disease occurrence, normally implemented on a computer. Such simulations may indicate which public health interventions are likely to be most effective or show where additional evidence needs to be acquired. Examples are models of the AIDS epidemic, screening programmes for cancer and carcinogenesis. A very early example – from 1760 – is Daniel Bernoulli's study on the effects of smallpox vaccination. We will not consider this branch any further.

Clinical

Clinical epidemiology is that part of the discipline applied to patients and clinical problems, rather than the population as a whole.

Concepts

The key concepts in epidemiology relate to risk. Risk is the probability of an event occurring. 'Risk' and 'probability' are used interchangeably. In a sample of individuals we can estimate risk of death as the proportion of individuals who die. We say that the number originally alive is the number 'at risk'.

$$\text{Risk} \quad = \quad \frac{\text{Deaths}}{\text{Population at risk}}$$

However, if 12 of a class of 30 school children die in 2 years, it is more worrying than if this occurred over 60 years. 'Rates' can be thought of as risk/unit time, so the denominator is person-time, which distinguishes a rate from a risk (typically this is expressed as x cases/100 000/year).

$$\text{Risk} \quad = \quad \frac{\text{Deaths}}{\text{Person-time at risk}}$$

'Person-time' is simply the sum of the times for which each individual in the population at risk is observed: one person living for 1 year equals 1 person-year. Two persons living for 6 months equals 1 person-year, one person living for 1 year plus one living for 2 years = 3 person-years. For population-level annual rates, the mid-year population estimate is used as an approximation.

For short periods and/or small risk, the rate approximates the risk. If the event is death (as above) this is termed a 'mortality rate'. If the event is a new diagnosis of disease, it is an 'incidence rate'. Incidence is simply the number of newly diagnosed cases in a given period. An 'age-specific rate' refers to a specific age group (for example, 35–39 year olds). Sex and social class-specific rates can be defined analogously.

'Odds' are another way of looking at risk. There is no mystery about odds and there is a one-to-one relationship between risk and odds:

$$\text{Odds} \quad = \quad \frac{\text{risk}}{(1 - \text{risk})}$$

We can easily convert odds to risk using:

$$\text{Risk} \quad = \quad \frac{\text{odds}}{(1 + \text{odds})}$$

Odds are sometimes more easily handled mathematically than risks. We can compare risks of disease in two groups using the ratio of the risks, the ratio of the rates or the ratio of the odds. Since these mathematically distinct measures are numerically very close for small risks, they are often referred to loosely as 'relative risk' – which strictly means just the risk ratio.

'Prevalence' is the number of cases alive with the disease either at a single point in time (point prevalence) or over a defined period (period prevalence). When these values are divided by the population size, we obtain so-called point and period prevalence 'rates' (actually not rates but proportions). If the duration of the disease and its incidence rate are not changing over time, then:

$$\text{Incidence rate} \times \text{Duration} = \text{Prevalence 'rate' (approximately)}$$

Descriptive epidemiology

The basic sources for descriptive epidemiology of disease are either *ad hoc* surveys or routinely available information in the form of official statistics published by the Office for National Statistics (ONS), formerly the Office of Population Censuses and Surveys (OPCS).

Population size is needed to obtain prevalence, incidence and mortality rates. This is obtained from the decennial Census. Between censuses, ONS provides the population estimates by subtracting deaths, adding births and allowing for emigrants, although these may be miscounted and the homeless may be missed.

Mortality

The registration of death has been compulsory since 1874 and mortality data tend to be of reasonably good quality (misclassification of death notwith-standing). Death certificates have an internationally agreed structure with Part I listing the immediate cause of death and conditions leading to it, from which the underlying cause is coded. Other significant conditions contribut-ing to the death are noted in Part II. The underlying cause is what appears in routine mortality statistics, but the other causes are coded at ONS.

For rapidly fatal diseases, the place and time of death is almost as good as place and time of diagnosis. Mortality data also offer complete population coverage, a clear end-point and long usage. Disadvantages are inaccuracy (in elderly people), an incomplete account of multiple pathology and inapplica-bility to nonfatal disease occurrence. Other important end-points such as quality of life and resource use are also missed.

Summarising mortality

When comparing disease mortality or incidence rates between different parts of the country, or between occupation groups, allowance needs to be made for variation in the age structure of the groups under study. Unadjusted rates are termed 'crude rates'. The effect of age can be allowed for by age-standard-isation, to yield 'age-adjusted' or 'age-standardised rates'.

There are two basic methods, direct and indirect standardisation but the details are not important here. The key point is that, as age varies with the groups under study and as the disease rate varies with age, this is basically a problem of confounding and standardisation is just another form of stratified analysis. Standardisation for sex and class is also possible.

Alternatives for mortality statistics are to present the cumulative risk of death from a disease ('lifetime' risk – actually to age 74 years) or to present a 'current life' table. This depicts what the survival of a single birth cohort would be if it experienced present-day mortality rates at each age.

Such life tables are used to estimate expectation of life from any age and are the basis for insurance, pension schemes and population forecasts. Variation between regions in expectation of life from birth has been shown to be greater than the effect of cancer.[1]

Male and female life tables for Trent are displayed in Figure 14.1 and show, for example, that median estimated survival from birth is about 5 years longer in women than men. English life tables are available in series DH1.

Morbidity

The most specific, accurate and complete routinely collected morbidity data are on cancer. The England and Wales National Cancer Registry, run by ONS, probably holds the largest registry data set on cancers in the world. It has

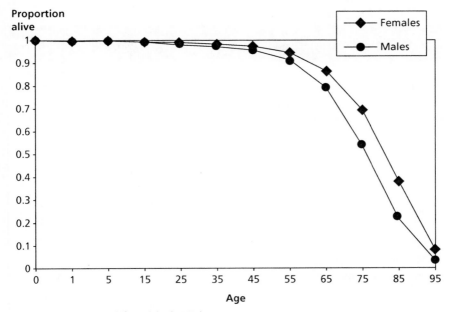

Figure 14.1   Trent life table (1991)

been estimated that the total data set now contains about 5 million cancers from a population of about 1500 million person-years at risk.

Cancer registration is not a statutory obligation. Data collection is organised through regional registries, which submit a standard data set to ONS. The origins of the system lie in hospital-based registries, which began in the 1920s. Since 1947, the General Register Office (now part of ONS) has taken on the responsibility.

The main disease-related routine statistics are listed in Table 14.1. Routinely available health-related information includes hospital episode statistics, the General Household Survey (questions on sickness-limited activity, visits to doctors and hospitals, and smoking and drinking habits), the National Food Survey (information on food purchases at regional level), and the Family Spending Survey (expenditure on food and tobacco).

A complete list of sources of routinely collected information is given in the *Guide to Official Statistics*.[2] Alternatively, visit the website: www.statistics.gov. uk. The Radical Statistics Group has issued a useful list and critique of sources of health statistics (see the reading list). Routine statistics delineate the north–south, urban–rural and social class variations in mortality, as well as being the basis for numerous descriptive and analytic epidemiological studies. Hospital episode statistics can be obtained from the Department of Health at www. dh.gov.uk/PublicationsAndStatistics/Statistics/HospitalEpisodeStatistics/ fs/en.

Table 14.1 Routinely available statistics on disease produced by the Office for National Statistics

Topic	Subset	Series
Vital statistics summary (population, births, deaths, fertility and mortality rates by region for England and Wales)		VS1
Mortality	General	DH1
	Cause	DH2
	Childhood, infant and perinatal	DH3
	Injury and poisoning	DH4
	Area*	DH5
Cancer registrations		MB1
Communicable disease		MB2
Congenital anomalies		MB3
General practice		MSGP4

*discontinued after 1992

Registers

A register is a database recording all cases of a disease (a form of event register) occurring in a defined population or recording all individuals exposed to a drug or procedure (an exposure register). A registry is the system or organisation that maintains the register. A good example of a disease register is the cancer registration system, which is clearly of value in assessing risks and outcomes of gynaecological malignancy or a birth defect register. An example of an exposure registry is the pregnancy register set up by a pharmaceutical company in order to study health effects of exposure to a particular medicine. Pregnancy registers may or may not include women who are not exposed to the medicine or procedure. Such studies are an example of phase V post-marketing studies and are set up either to describe the current state of affairs and generate hypotheses or to examine issues that are not susceptible to study in an RCT, using cohort or case–control methods. Unlike the cancer registries, which are funded on a 'permanent' basis, the exposure registries tend to have a finite life.

Analytic epidemiology

Aetiology

We actually observe only the conjunction of events, from which we must infer cause. This is easy when events occur together almost universally or when they are under our direct voluntary control. More generally, we have to extend the concept of cause to events that are only 'probable', by looking for association. Association is when events occur together more, or less, often than one would expect. In epidemiology, association is typically measured by:

- the difference in risk of disease between exposed and unexposed (excess risk)
- the ratio of the risk in exposed to the risk in unexposed (relative risk)
- the ratio of the odds of disease in exposed to the odds in unexposed (odds ratio).

If no association is present the excess risk will be 0 and the relative risk (and odds ratio) will be 1. The difficulty lies in determining whether an association is causal (recognising that most diseases are multifactorial and that causes may operate by predisposing an individual to a disease, precipitating its onset or aggravating its course). Pragmatic criteria for accepting an association as causal in observational studies were suggested by Bradford Hill:[3]

- consistency of association – results are replicated in studies using different methods, in a variety of settings
- strength of association – the larger the magnitude of the excess risk or relative risk the more persuasive the evidence
- specificity – when a suspected cause produces a single well-defined effect

- dose–response relationship – when increasing the exposure produces larger excess or relative risks
- time sequence – the exposure must have preceded the event
- biological plausibility – when the association makes biological sense
- coherence – for example if the association 'explains' other facts known about the disease, such as age and sex distribution
- experiment – if removal of the cause reduces the risk of disease.

Ways of establishing association

We can do this by means of intervention studies (experiment, including RCTs) or by observational studies, using either the traditional cohort or the case–control approach or one of the newer case-only designs. For any of these, the units or subjects of study may be at an ecological or individual level.

An example of an ecological level observational study is the correlation of breast cancer mortality rates and average fat consumption in different countries. For intervention studies, an example would be the reduction in cervical cancer mortality rates following the introduction of a screening programme. Ecological level studies also arise in the context of RCTs as 'cluster randomised' studies.

The weakness of ecological level studies is that associations found at group level need not appear when individuals are studied. This is called the ecologic fallacy. Ecological level studies are useful to generate hypotheses, and are appropriate if the proposed intervention will be applied anyway in a mass fashion (such as legislation).

The RCT is probably the kind of intervention study most familiar to clinicians, and can be illustrated as follows:

- Aim: does ovarian cancer respond better to Taxol® than to conventional chemotherapy?
- Method: choose suitable patients, randomise to Taxol® and control groups, measure percentage responding.
- Result: Taxol group has greater percentage of responders (or not).

The key point is that subjects are alike, apart from the exposure of interest. The cohort study is basically the same except that, crucially, allocation to the exposure is no longer under the investigator's control:

- Aim: does smoking cause cervical cancer?
- Method: choose subjects without cervical cancer, identify smokers and non-smokers, follow them over time.
- Result: greater percentage of cervical cancer cases in smokers (maybe).

Both the RCT and the cohort study can be depicted in a 2 × 2 table (Table 14.2). In practice, the results are likely to be expressed as rates rather than risks, with person-time as the denominator but, as rates can be converted to risks and hence odds, this does not affect the argument. Case–control studies appear at first sight to be different, since the answer to the smoking question is obtained in a 'back to front' manner and the probabilities of previous exposure are compared, not the risks of getting the disease:

- Aim: does smoking cause cervical cancer?
- Method: choose subjects, identify cervical cancer cases and controls (without cervical cancer), ask about past smoking.
- Result: greater percentage of smokers in cervical cancer patients.

However, looking at the corresponding 2 × 2 table (Table 14.3), it can be seen that the relative odds of exposure are the same as the relative odds of disease which would have been obtained from a cohort study (provided the disease was rare). Thus, while the case–control study cannot estimate relative risk directly (you sample cases and controls), provided the disease is rare, the odds ratio you obtain from a case–control study numerically approximates the relative risk you would have obtained from a cohort.

In fact, what the case–control study estimates depends on how the controls are chosen. If the case–control study is regarded as a way of economically analysing a cohort, then the relative risk is estimated by setting up the case–control study so that controls are chosen at random (with a known probability) from all individuals who are at risk at the beginning of the study, including those who eventually become cases. This is called a 'case-base' study. If controls are chosen from the pool of those who are disease-free at the time a case occurs, so that controls for one case may subsequently become cases themselves (a 'case-cohort' study) then the hazard ratio (relative rate) is estimated: the same mathematics applying as in Cox regression, as seen in Figure 14.2.

Table 14.2 Randomised controlled trials and cohort studies

	Become ill	Do not become ill
Exposed	a	b
Unexposed	c	d
Total	a + b	c + d

$$\text{Relative risk of disease} = \frac{a/(a+b)}{c/(c+d)} \approx \frac{ad}{bc} \quad \text{if the disease is rare (when } a<<b, \text{ and } c<<d)$$

Table 14.3 Case–control studies

	Become ill	Do not become ill
Exposed	a	b
Unexposed	c	d
Total	a+c	b+d

$$\text{Relative odds of exposure} = \frac{a/c}{b/d} \approx \frac{ad}{bc}$$

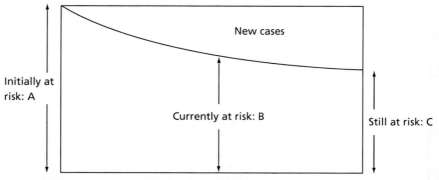

Figure 14.2   Choice of controls affects what a case–control study measures: exposure odds ratio measures risk ratio if controls are sampled at A, rate ratio if controls are sampled at B, disease odds ratio if controls are sampled at C (adapted from Rodrigues and Kirkwood, 1990)[32]

You may also come across cohort studies in which usually the mortality rate is compared with that expected from the general population. If 'O' is the number of observed deaths and 'E' the number expected number of deaths, taking into account the age and sex structure of the exposed group, then the standardised mortality ratio, or SMR (= O/E), is also the relative risk in the exposed group compared with the general population. This will be close to the relative risk of exposed to unexposed if exposure is rare in the general population.

Historical cohort studies use existing records to reconstruct exposures histories that occurred in the possibly distant past and with determination of the subsequent outcome. This approach can be especially useful for studies of occupational exposure: for example, comparing subsequent incidence of mesothelioma and ovarian cancer in women exposed to asbestos while working as gas mask assemblers.[4] The method was also used in studies of birth weight and subsequent development of cardiovascular disease.[5] Such studies are now impeded by laws on data protection and requirements for consent.

The results of a case–control and a cohort study on the effects of smoking are shown in Tables 14.4[6] and 14.5[7], respectively. In Table 14.4, note the high prevalence of smoking among the controls. This reflects (a) the high prevalence of smoking in men at that time and (b) some degree of selection bias in that controls were hospital patients. Note the similarity of the three measures of 'relative risk' in Table 14.5 because annual risk is small.

Case-only designs are not to be confused with case-series. They can be summarised as case only, case-crossover, matched cohort, case–time–control.[8] The motivation of the case-crossover design is like that for a crossover RCT. In its simplest form, the exposure to a risk factor during the period in which an individual experienced an event is compared with the exposure during a matched period in which the event did not occur – the analysis being like that of a matched

Table 14.4 Case–control study: cigarettes and lung cancer, males[6]

	Cases	Controls
Smoker	1350	1296
Non-smoker	7	61

$$\frac{\text{Relative odds}}{\text{(odds ratio)}} = \frac{1350/7}{1296/61} \approx \frac{1350 \times 61}{1296 \times 7} = 9$$

Table 14.5 Cohort study: cigarettes and lung cancer (adapted from Hammond and Horn)[7]

	Lung cancer deaths	Person-years at risk	Rate/ year	Annual risk	Annual odds
Cigarette smokers	249	195 754.7	0.001272	0.001271	0.001271
Non-smokers	15	117 187.5	0.000128	0.000128	0.000128
Rate ratio	9.938				
Risk ratio	9.932				
Odds ratio	9.930				

case–control study. Assumptions of this design are: brief exposure, quick effect, acute, recognisable illness and no carry-over of exposure effect from one period to the next. This design is good for assessing precipitating factors of disease and applications have included study of triggers of myocardial infarction and the relation between mobile phone use while driving and car accidents. A good description is given by Maclure.[9] Advantages are that it is cheap (half the size of case–control study, as it only need cases and each gives multiple controls), and it does not need information on confounders – it is matched.

In the matched cohort design, each exposed individual is matched to one or more unexposed one. Finding the matches can be time consuming and wastes unmatched subjects; moreover, the association of outcome with the matching variable cannot be studied. In general, cohort studies tend not to be matched nowadays. However, with matched cohort designs, the matched sets in which no one experiences the outcome do not actually contribute any information about the relative risk. If the data collection can be organised so that only individuals known to have experienced the event are studied, this can offer a large saving in resources. For example, in the study on vasectomy and risk of heart attack conducted by Walker et al.,[10] in only 36 of 4830 matched pairs did at least one subject have a heart attack, so case notes for other confounding variables only needed to be examined for these 72 subjects. Another suitable application is when matching can be done within persons, for example in studies of the occurrence of fits following vaccination), where the model was described as a self-controlled case series.[11] A good description is given by Cummings et al.[12]

Lastly, the case–time–control design may be thought of as a hybrid between a case–control and a case-crossover design. Basically, two parallel studies are set up, a case-crossover design and a 'control-crossover' design, the controls being matched to the cases in the usual way. The odds ratio from the case-crossover analysis is then 'corrected' by odds ratio from control-crossover, the intention being to adjust for any time trends occurring in exposure.

The approach to use depends on circumstances. Intervention studies raise ethical issues if subjects will be deliberately exposed to harm but do ensure that time sequence is met and that intervention and control groups are alike apart from the exposure. Case–control studies allow many possible exposures to be evaluated for one disease but measurement of past exposure can be difficult and cases may be hard to find unless concentrated, in a hospital, for example. Cohort studies allow the study of many different consequences from a single kind of exposure but if exposure is rare the cohort may be hard to assemble and adequate follow-up may be a problem. Case-only designs are good for explaining 'why this patient developed this disease now' but involve extra assumptions about exposure effects.

Relative risk measures association but we need to know about absolute risks too, because a large relative increase from a small baseline risk may not be as bad as a small relative increase from a high baseline. Cohort studies do automatically give absolute risk; case–control studies will only do this if designed to sample incident cases from a defined population and time period.

Confounding

The weakness of observational studies is lack of control over additional factors associated both with exposure and outcome. The result may be a spurious association (or its lack) between two variables, due to their mutual association with a third, confounding variable. For example, the risk of lung cancer is greater in manual workers but this is largely due to the fact that they are more likely to smoke and smoking is associated with lung cancer, as shown in Figure 14.3. How can we deal with confounding?

- think of it
- measure/record the presence of the confounder during the study
- allow for it in the analysis.

There is no great mystery – essentially, it is a matter of comparing like with like. The possibilities are:

- stratification
- matching
- statistical modelling.

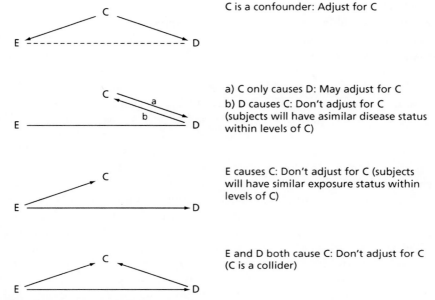

C is a confounder: Adjust for C

a) C only causes D: May adjust for C
b) D causes C: Don't adjust for C
(subjects will have asimilar disease status
within levels of C)

E causes C: Don't adjust for C (subjects
will have similar exposure status within
levels of C)

E and D both cause C: Don't adjust for C
(C is a collider)

Figure 14.3 Do we adjust or not?

Stratification
Group subjects into strata according to predefined characteristics such as age
group, sex, disease severity.

Matching
Matching is an extreme form of stratification where each stratum is often just
two subjects; for example, a case–control pair. More than two controls may be
chosen per case and the number of controls does not have to be the same for
each case. These very fine strata are termed matched sets. Matching is also
possible in RCTs.

Statistical modelling
This is the modern approach, heavily dependent on computers. While it may
seem forbidding, there is no alternative if you are to benefit fully from modern
statistical methods. In practice, Windows-based systems such as SPSS,
StatsDirect or MINITAB are easy to operate and statistics textbooks exist
that refer to such packages.

Multiple logistic regression is used for case–control studies and models
the odds of being a case, using a multiple regression-like formula:

$$\log(P/(1 - P)) = b_0 + b_1 x_1 + b_2 x_2$$

The right-hand side of the equation is called a linear predictor. The variables
might be categories; thus it would be allowed to have $b_3\, x(\text{sex})$ if sex was

coded as 0 = male, 1 = female. The variable coding for sex is called a dummy or indicator variable. The position is a little more elaborate if there are more than two categories (for example, if race was to be allowed for). In this case separate dummy variables have to be created for one less than the number of categories.

The odds ratio for variable x_1 adjusted for the other factors is $\exp(b_1)$. Conditional logistic regression is a special variant for matched case–control studies. It is better than a conventional matched analysis because it is possible to match on one or two key variables, and model the effects of others.

Poisson regression does the same for cohort studies, this time modelling the disease rate, and is closely linked with Cox regression (used in survival analysis and applied in RCTs and studies of prognosis).

The purpose of stratified and matched analyses is to remove or 'adjust for' the effect of a confounding variable: the variable(s) defining the strata or matched set. The effect of treatment or exposure is assessed within strata and a single overall 'adjusted' figure is obtained by averaging over the strata.

Modelling effectively does the same but it is more flexible because you can look for joint effects/interactions very easily. Moreover, matching is expensive (it can be hard to find matches when you are matching on several variables) and unnecessary matching (on variables that are not confounders) is inefficient, giving wider confidence limits (CL).

You especially should not adjust for colliders, as shown in Figure 14.3, because this will induce a spurious association between E and D. Why is this? It is simple: imagine E, C and D each have only two levels, high and low. If E and D both cause C then for high levels of C, E and D will both tend to be high, while for low levels of C, both E and D will tend to be low; in other words D and E will be correlated with each other within each stratum of C but this is purely an artefact. Adjustment by matching, stratification or modelling will give an incorrect result.

It is now widely recognised that statistics cannot substitute for *a priori* causal knowledge in deciding which variables are confounders. Do not use statistical tests or less formal methods (for example, seeing if the unadjusted analysis differs materially from the unadjusted one) to decide whether a variable is a confounder or not.

Effect modification

Some variables can alter the effect of an exposure; for example, prior immunisation will modify the risk of developing disease, given exposure. That is, there is an interaction between the effect modifier and the exposure. This is distinct from confounding because the effect will arise even if the exposure is equally distributed across categories of the effect modifier. Again, modelling can detect such effects easily by representing interactions as a product of the variables concerned.

Bias

All studies are potentially subject to bias: a systematic deviation from the truth. Unlike confounding it cannot be dealt with by statistical analysis. The effect is that 'like is no longer compared with like'. Bias can arise when:

- selecting subjects for a study
- allocating them to treatments
- measuring exposure
- attempting follow-up
- analysing and presenting results.

The main protection is to think of the possibility and design it out. Possible strategies include:

- random sampling in surveys
- randomised allocation in intervention studies
- objective rather than subjective endpoints
- blinded (masked) assessment and analysis
- high participation
- no missing data
- low drop out (to obtain these final three requires persistence and persuasion).

How much disease is 'due to' a given cause?

The aetiological fraction (also called population attributable risk) is the proportion of cases of a disease 'due to' a risk factor; it is often expressed as a percentage. For cohort studies, it can be estimated from the formula:

$$\frac{[\text{Total incidence rate in population} - \text{Incidence rate in unexposed}]}{\text{Total incidence rate in population}}$$

However, it is not possible to apply this to the Hammond and Horn[7] data in Table 14.5 because the table omits results for other types of tobacco. For case–control studies, a different formula is used (derived from the one above), which emphasises that the impact on a population depends on the proportion exposed as well as the relative increase in risk:

Aetiological fraction (population attributable risk) $= p(R-1)/[p(R-1) + 1]$

where p = proportion of population exposed to risk factor,
R = odds ratio of disease, given exposure.

For example, if 30% of men smoke ($p = 0.3$), $R = 14$, aetiological fraction is 80%. We also see that even if everyone was exposed ($p = 1$) then the proportion of cases still unexplained by the exposure would be about 7%:

$$1 - (R - 1)/R$$

Diagnosis

The first problem is what do we mean by 'a case' of a disease? Epidemiologists tend to use one of the following criteria:

- Oddity (in a statistical sense), when a measured value is unusually low or high: if we set an arbitrary cut-off point (for example, 5th and 95th centiles) then a constant fraction of the population will be 'ill' and this definition need not bear any relation to symptoms.
- Risk: someone is not considered diseased until they have a 'high' risk of some consequence, such as serum uric acid and risk of gout. But where do we draw the line?
- Cut-offs: are not easy to define when risk increases linearly.
- Illness: however, this may exclude many people who could benefit from treatment even though they have no symptoms at present – this is the idea behind screening for cancer, for example.
- Better off: the question now is whether the possibly adverse consequences of treatment outweigh the consequences of not treating the condition: removing skin moles can leave a scar; we accept this risk when we consider that there is a substantial risk of melanoma.

We infer that a patient has a disease by applying tests. The aim is to distinguish people with the disease from those without. This is an instance of the more general problem of classification. The basic idea of a diagnostic test is that the likelihood of having the disease is related to the level of some measurable characteristic. Levels of this above a threshold value are termed positive and indicate the presence of disease.

Tests may be pathognomic (defining the condition) and form a gold standard against which other, surrogate, tests may be compared. Surrogate tests measure a proxy variable for the condition with which we are really concerned; clearly, all screening tests use proxy variables but, in fact, the results of most familiar medical investigations such as serology for hepatitis B or creatine kinase for myocardial infarction are surrogates for the actual presence of disease. Surrogate tests are used when they are cheaper, simpler, safer or more acceptable than pathognomonic tests. These issues are especially important in screening as it is concerned with the routine search for asymptomatic disease.

Where a pathognomic test is hard to define, tests may be evaluated relative to some other surrogate or to the results of a combination of surrogate tests. Any good diagnostic test will be accurate (or valid) and repeatable.

Accuracy (validity)

For continuous variables, such as blood glucose, we must define the threshold for a positive diagnosis. Given this threshold, we can evaluate the test in terms of:

- sensitivity = proportion of diseased who test positive
- specificity = proportion of non-diseased who test negative.

Suppose we want to detect impaired glucose tolerance using venous blood taken two hours after a 75 g oral glucose challenge. The results from a sample of known diabetics and a sample of non-diabetics might look like those in Table 14.6, using a cut-point of 7.8 mmol/l above which a test is 'positive'; which gives a sensitivity of 74% and specificity of 91%. Why choose 7.8 mmol/l; why not 6.1 or 8.3? At the best (most discriminating) cut-off point the difference between sensitivity and (1– specificity) will be greatest (Table 14.7).

The receiver operating characteristic (ROC) plot is a graphical way to find the optimum and a way of displaying the performance of the test over a range of cut-off points. For detecting impaired glucose tolerance, an ROC plot might look like that in Figure 14.4 (the results of useless, non-discriminating, tests will lie on the 'line of identity').

Similar analyses can be applied to find the most discriminating cut-off point for ordered categories, such as abnormalities found on cervical cytology.

Summarising test performance

Test performance is measured by the area under the ROC curve (AUC). A useless test gives a value of 0.5 but the data for the impaired glucose tolerance gave an AUC of 0.88 (95% confidence limits 0.82–0.94).

Probability of disease given a test result

We need to know the prevalence, p, of the condition in the population tested (the prevalence is likely to be higher in a hospital outpatient clinic than in a GP's surgery). The prevalence is the probability prior to the test result of

Table 14.6 Sensitivity and specificity		
Blood glucose test result	Diabetics	Non-diabetics
Positive (> 7.8 mmol/l)	74	9
Negative (≤ 7.8 mmol/l)	26	91
Total	100	100

Sensitivity = proportion of diabetics who test positive = 74/100 = 0.74
Specificity = proportion of non-diabetics who test negative = 91/100 = 0.91

Table 14.7 Good and bad discrimination				
Test	(a) A test with good discrimination		(b) A test with poor discrimination	
	Diseased	Non-diseased	Diseased	Non-diseased
Positive	90	1	90	90
Negative	10	99	10	10
Total	100	100	100	100
Sensitivity – (1 – specificity) = 0.89			Sensitivity – (1 – specificity) = 0	

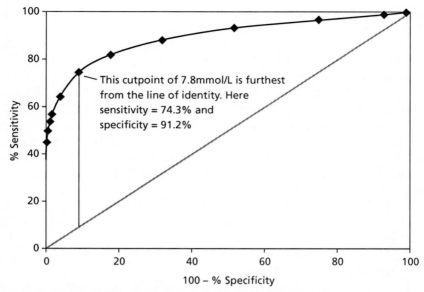

Figure 14.4 The ROC plot (2-hour postprandial blood glucose)

having the disease (hence prior probability). We must also combine sensitivity and specificity in a single index:

$$\text{The Likelihood ratio for a positive test} = \frac{\text{Sensitivity}}{(1 - \text{Specificity})}$$

The steps are:
- Convert this to prior odds using odds = $p/(1-p)$; that is, the odds of someone chosen 'at random' being diseased.

The Posterior odds are the odds that someone chosen 'at random is diseased', when they have tested positive:

$$\text{Posterior odds} = \text{Prior odds} \times \text{Likelihood ratio of a positive test}$$

- Convert the odds back to the probability of being diseased, given a positive test result (posterior probability):

$$\text{Probability of disease given a positive test} = \frac{\text{Posterior odds}}{(1 + \text{Posterior odds})}$$

This is also called the (positive) predictive value of a positive test.

We can define the odds of not being diseased given a negative test too:

$$\text{Prior odds of health} \times \frac{\text{Specificity}}{(1 - \text{Sensitivity})}$$

Note that the interpretation of the result of a test depends on how common the disease is in the first place ('common things occur commonly'). If prevalence is high, a negative result will not convincingly rule out the diagnosis. Conversely, a positive result will not be overwhelming evidence for the disease if prevalence is low. For example, if the prevalence of disease is 64%, with a test sensitivity of 74.3% and specificity of 91.2%, although the probability of disease given a positive test is 94%, there is still a 33% chance of being diseased if the test result is negative. In practice, for most diseases, the prior probability will not be enormously high until several investigations have been positive.

The thing to remember is that, in general, high sensitivity rules out the disease, for example, ERCP for pancreatic cancer: 'if negative, chances are good'. Conversely, high specificity, for example, liver biopsy for secondary cancer, is not sensitive but 'if positive it's definite'. Sackett et al.[13] use the mnemonic 'SnOUT and SpIN'.

Repeatability

This is the extent to which diagnoses or other measurements agree from occasion to occasion. Typical concerns are the extent to which:

- a single observer's diagnoses are self-consistent (evaluated on different occasions but using the same observer and patients)
- the diagnoses made by several observers are mutually consistent (typically evaluated using a panel of observers on a single set of patients).

For interval or ratio scale data, the appropriate index is an intra-class correlation coefficient found using components of variance. This indicates how much of the overall variation in a set of measurements is due to between-patient variation rather than variation in the measurement process itself (disagreement).

For nominal scales, the corresponding index is the κ (kappa) statistic. This is the proportion of cases for whom two observers agree a diagnosis, correcting for the agreement to be expected by chance. If a panel of observers is used, κ measures the average pairwise agreement. When only two diagnoses are possible, κ can be shown to be effectively an intra-class correlation and for three or more diagnoses, the overall κ is an average of the κ produced for each category versus the others combined. The idea can be extended to give a κ even when not all the observers in a panel assess every patient (Table 14.8). In fact, despite their apparent dissimilarity, both κ and intra-class correlation

Table 14.8	Example of κ – two pathologists compared assessments of cervical biopsies[14]				
First observer's opinion	**Second observer's opinion**				
	Invasive carcinoma	**In situ carcinoma**	**Severe dysplasia**	**Normal/mild dysplasia**	**Total**
Invasive carcinoma	11	0	0	0	11
In situ carcinoma	2	13	0	0	15
Severe dysplasia	0	6	22	1	29
Normal/mild dysplasia	0	1	3	19	23
Total	13	20	25	20	78

Observed proportion of agreements = (11 + 13 + 22 + 19)/78 = 0.83

Chance-expected proportion = (13 × 11/78 + 20 × 15/78 + 25 × 29/78 + 20 × 23/78)/78 = 0.27

NB the expected numbers are found as in a χ^2 test as (row total × column total/grand total). These are added and divided again by the grand total to get the expected proportion of agreement

κ = (Observed proportion – Expected proportion)/(1 – Expected proportion) = (0.83 – 0.27)/(1 – 0.27) = 0.77

coefficients are instances of a reliability coefficient and can be recast in the general form of:

$$\text{Reliability} = 1 - \left[\frac{\text{observed errors}}{\text{chance} - \text{expected errors}} \right]$$

While κ (and intra-class correlations) correct for chance-expected agreement in a given sample of patients and observers, they are affected by the case-mix so that a sample of patients drawn from a different population may give a different κ even if nothing else has changed. This is called the base rate problem and means that κ values are not comparable between different studies unless the proportions of each diagnostic category are similar. For example, suppose we have two observers and three tumour types: 'squamous carcinoma', 'adenocarcinoma' and 'other' and the probabilities of agreement given each tumour type are fixed. A case mix of: 33 squamous, 33 adeno, 34 other gives a $\kappa = 0.55$ with standard error of 0.069. However, a case mix of 56 squamous, 29 adeno, 15 other gives a $\kappa = 0.46$ with standard error of 0.081, so case-mix affects both κ and its confidence limits.

κ ranges from 1 (indicating perfect agreement) through 0 (indicating agreement no better than by chance) to negative values (indicating disagreement beyond chance expectation). There is no fixed lower limit for κ, unlike an intra-class correlation, which ranges from 0 to 1.

What are 'good values'? Landis and Koch[15] gave the following benchmarks:

- < 0 .01 'poor'
- 0.01–0.20 'slight'
- 0.21–0.40 'fair'
- 0.41–0.60 'moderate'
- 0.61–0.80 'substantial'
- > 0.80 'almost perfect'.

However, these need to be interpreted relative to what is needed, what it is reasonable to expect and what is possible given the prevalence of each disease category. In practice, typical values can be disappointingly low. For subtypes of non-small-cell lung cancer between-observer κ in one study was only 0.39; similar agreement (between-observer κ of 0.44) has been found on the presence of cholestasis-plugs in liver biopsies, although within-observer κ was 0.766 indicating self-consistency, at least.[16]

A refinement is weighted κ, which takes into account the relative importance of each type of disagreement. For example, if one observer diagnoses '*in situ* carcinoma' and the other, 'invasive carcinoma', this is much less serious than if one diagnoses 'normal' and the other 'invasive carcinoma'. Weighted κ is most suitable for ordered categories (as in the example above) but even then a generally accepted set of weights for each disagreement may not be feasible. If the data really lie on an interval scale, then it would be better to use an intra-class correlation. Agreement studies can be improved by:

- standardising measurement conditions
- training to a uniform level of competence
- using objective measurements
- ensuring patients are representative in terms of range and severity of conditions.

Possible applications are to:

- prove comparable performance in assessing patients for RCTs
- demonstrate adequate repeatability for screening programmes
- identify repeatable classifications prior to validation in terms of sensitivity/specificity
- help simplify diagnostic classifications
- identify 'cliques' of observers (whose diagnoses tend to be similar).

Prognosis
A prognosis is simply a forecast, or prediction, of the course or outcome of a disease. Characteristics which influence outcome may be summarised in a cause-and-effect diagram, such as Figure 14.5, which summarises factors affecting survival time in cancer. Typically, prognostic factors, as such, are taken to be properties of the disease state or the patient but we can extend the concept to include treatment-related factors as well. Because the forecast is an estimate of what will happen, based on experience with similar individuals in

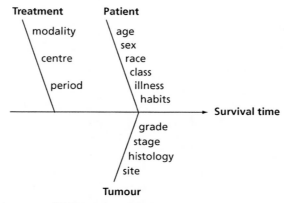

Figure 14.5 Factors affecting prognosis

the past, there has to be some uncertainty about the result. For an individual patient, the forecast result may not happen: it can only be 'statistical'. This does not mean that the method used to produce the forecast is wrong, because the forecast only predicts what will happen on average. It is, therefore, most important to realise that confidence limits on the mean survival time, for example, reflect uncertainty about the estimate of the mean and not the variability in individual patient survival.

A classic form of outcome is death or occurrence of complications. We may extend this by measuring time to the event. This clearly applies to survival from a disease but also applies to time of first occurrence (of a multiple event such as a migraine attack) and survival analysis methods can equally be used for any other non-negative quantity, not necessarily time at all. Such results can be presented graphically in a survival plot, which displays the proportion of the original subjects remaining alive against time since diagnosis, as shown in Figure 14.6.

The y axis in Figure 14.6 indicates $S(t)$ – the proportion of survivors at time t, while t itself is shown on the x axis.

We can use such a plot to read off the median survival or the proportion alive at any given time (the same as the proportion living at least that time). The 'steps' come about because of the way the plot is estimated: survival is constant until someone dies and then it jumps. As the sample size increases, the plot progressively approaches a smooth curve. Modern packages will construct plots automatically given survival times.

Censoring and withdrawal

One peculiarity of survival data is that survival times may be censored. Imagine 100 patients followed from diagnosis until 2 years have elapsed. The naïve way to produce a survival plot would be to plot each month the number still alive/100. This survival plot would be straightforward but suppose a newly diagnosed patient joined the group after the study had been running

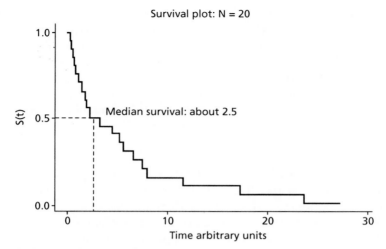

Figure 14.6 Typical survival plot

for 18 months and was still alive 6 months after diagnosis when follow-up ceased? We say such an observation is censored, as we know the patient lived at least 6 months but the exact time survived is unknown. Another way in which censored survival times occur is if patients move away during the 2 years and are lost to follow-up. Provided that this occurs at random, we can treat such cases the same way as if censored owing to the end of the study period. Because of this peculiarity, in practice, survival plots are not constructed using the number remaining alive but are produced indirectly, using the hazard (it is the instantaneous probability of dying). For each moment in time:

$$\text{Hazard} = h(t) = \frac{\text{Deaths}}{(\text{Number at risk at time } t)}$$

At each time point, if no patient dies the hazard is 0 and if patients are censored they reduce only the denominator. We then have:

$S(t)$ = Probability of surviving to at least t
    = Probability of surviving each interval to t
    = $(1 - h_1)(1 - h_2)...(1 - h_t)$ where h_1
    = hazard from time 0 to t_1, h_2
    = hazard from time t_1 to time t_2 and ht
    = hazard over the final interval up to time t (all the intervals being
    vanishingly small).

This estimate is the Kaplan–Meier estimator of $S(t)$. If values are given rather than plotted, it is a form of life table.

Comparing two or more survival curves is essentially a matter of comparing hazards at each time. The most common method effectively averages the hazard ratios and calculates a form of chi-square statistic on the observed number of deaths compared with that expected if the average hazard ratio over time were 1. This is the log-rank test.

Cox regression models the hazard ratio in a multiple regression-like way, allowing for the effect of many variables to be incorporated:

$$\log(RR) = b_1x_1 + b_2x_2 + \dots$$

As exp(b) gives the relative risk, if $b > 0$ the corresponding variable increases the risk (shortens survival). If there is more than one variable, exponentiating one coefficient gives the relative risk for that variable, having adjusted for the presence of all the other predictor variables in the equation. Exponentiating the whole linear predictor for a given combination of values gives the total relative risk for that combination.

Forming prognostic groups, validation and discriminatory power

We can form prognostic groups from the distribution of values of the linear predictor. For example, we might define 'good', 'intermediate' and 'poor' prognostic groups by using the lower and upper tertiles of the linear predictor as cut-off points. Note that, since the greater the value of the linear predictor the greater the risk of dying, a high value for the linear predictor is bad news. The linear predictor can now be used directly as a prognostic index. Often, it is a simplified version of the original linear predictor; for example, coefficients may be rounded to the nearest integer.

Once a prognostic index has been constructed for a set of patients, its performance needs to be validated in terms of how well it discriminates between patients 'who do well' and those who do not. In general, a prognostic index will not perform so well on a second or subsequent sets of patients, because it will have been tailored to the original 'training set'. The actual performance can be estimated in a number of ways; one is to have a separate 'validation' set of patients; that is, the prognostic index is cross-validated.

Another way to construct prognostic groups is by constructing a decision tree (also called a classification or regression tree). A variety of software exists for this – perhaps the best known being CART™. The advantages of trees are that they are readily understood on visual inspection, lend themselves easily to clinical algorithms and are usable with missing data (for a patient with some variables missing you only progress down the tree as far as you have complete data). On the other hand, they are less well placed to assess the magnitude of the joint effects of different variables. Another difference between a prognostic index and a decision tree like that developed by CART is that the decision tree automatically generates the prognostic groups identified from the data whereas groups based on the prognostic index must be defined arbitrarily, for example by splitting at the quartiles of the index. On the other hand, with a prognostic index the groups can be defined so as to have equal numbers.

How is the performance of the prognostic index to be measured? One suggestion is to use a rank-based measure of concordance between rankings on the prognostic index and the survival time. The result is a proportion of concordant rankings that can be thought of as a generalisation of the area under an ROC curve.

Case-fatality 'rate' is another measure of outcome, especially useful when the disease is brief, as in plague, cholera or meningitis. It is defined as:

$$\frac{\text{Number of deaths from a disease in a given period} \times 100\%}{\text{Number of new cases of the disease in the same period}}$$

This can lead to problems when more people die of the disease in a given period than develop it. For example, in Trent region during 1990, 173 women aged 85 years or older died of breast cancer whereas only 140 women developed the disease. The problem of course is that the deaths occur over a period of several years, well after the onset of the disease. It is better to use a different definition, based on the survival curve of patients followed from the point of diagnosis. However we can also use the survival curve to answer a slightly different question, namely that of 'cure'.

Can we tell if 'cure' is possible? Often, we would like an estimate of the proportion of people who are cured of a disease such as cancer; in effect, this is the complement of the case-fatality rate mentioned earlier. Some cancers, such as those of the pancreas, kill virtually all patients within 1 or 2 years, whereas breast cancers have relatively good survival rate, although even 20 years later the patient may develop a recurrence and die. In general, we cannot be sure that an individual has been cured. We can, however, define a 'statistical

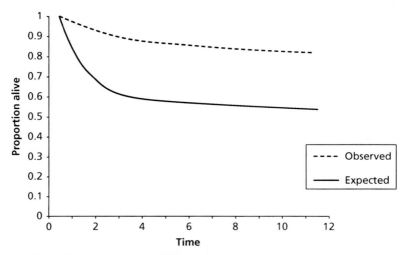

Figure 14.7   Observed and expected survival

cure', applied to a group of people, which can be used as the probability that an individual will be cured.

Demonstration of a statistical cure can be seen graphically, as in Figure 14.7. The solid line denotes the expected percentage survival at each time after diagnosis, while the dashed line is the observed percentage survival.

If we plot relative survival (observed/expected) against time, then when the plot becomes constant, it can be shown algebraically that at this point the annual death rate from all causes is similar to that of a normal population of the same age and sex distribution. We say that this group shows statistical evidence of a cure and the fraction cured is given by the relative survival at the time the plot becomes constant. In the example depicted in Figure 14.8, it is about 68%. In essence, this assesses the effect of therapy on the excess mortality due the disease.

Such statistical cure seems to have been demonstrated for some cancers (for example childhood leukaemia) but not others (such as breast cancer). Some difficulties are that a long follow-up is required, to be sure that 'cure' is reached but, by then, the numbers at risk are relatively small; hence, there is in practice a question of sampling error. Also, during a long follow-up a new treatment may have changed things (such as penicillin). Moreover, it is important to use the right sort of comparison group: mortality rates should be derived from the same area that has supplied the patients and ideally be comparable with respect to other factors (for example, smoking, social status and length of residence) that affect death rates. This is hardly ever possible. Lastly, as time goes by, the relative survival curve tends to be weighted towards that of the younger members of the cohort of patients, who by now predominate, giving a falsely optimistic picture of the possibility of cure.

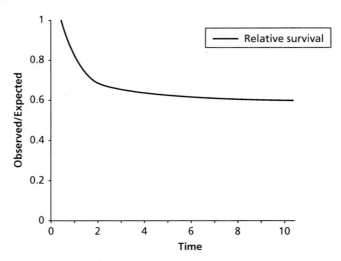

Figure 14.8 Relative survival

Other forms of outcome

Outcome need not be assessed on an 'all or none' scale or restricted to survival. They may be measurable on an ordinal scale, such as morbidity or pain, or measurable on an interval scale, such as blood pressure, CD4 lymphocyte count or FEV_1. It is important to know, however, whether these are an end in themselves or whether they are a surrogate for some other measure, such as survival time. Be wary of surrogate outcomes. Bear in mind that these are a substitute for the quantity you really want to measure, such as how a patient feels, functions or survives. Surrogates may be considered when direct measurement of a clinically relevant effect is too hard, too costly or too time consuming. However, for use of the surrogate to be justified:

- there should be biological plausibility of the relationship with clinical outcome
- observational studies must have shown the surrogate has strong prognostic value, after adjusting for confounders
- RCTs must show that effects of treatment on surrogate correspond to effects on clinical outcome
- there should be consistency across studies.

Problems with surrogates are that they may not reflect the full range of effects, there may not be a quantitative measure of benefit for comparison with risks, a one-to-one relation with clinical outcome is very unlikely and the surrogate may not work for other interventions. If an indicator such as 'quality of life' is measured several times during the course of an illness, it might look like that in Figure 14.9.

We can combine 'quality of life' and survival by multiplying each year a patient survives by the 'quality of life' experienced, possibly including a

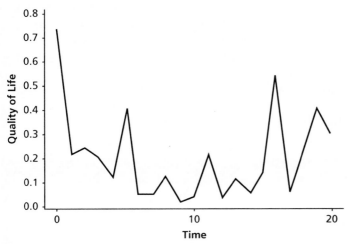

Figure 14.9 Quality of life for a single patient (hypothetical)

'discount' factor. The result is the 'quality adjusted life-year' or QALY often used in determining treatment policies.

Other topics in epidemiology

Capture–recapture

These methods (also called capture–mark–recapture) have been used in eco-logical studies to estimate fish stocks, in clinical practice to estimate the true prevalence of diabetes and in cancer registries to estimate the completeness of ascertainment. In fact, in its simplest form the method is also related to the dilution techniques used to estimate the volume of body compartments. In animal population studies, a sample of animals is trapped, marked and released. A second sample is obtained by setting another set of traps and the number of marked animals and unmarked animals in the second sample is recorded. Suppose we have two incomplete lists of patients with a particular condition, drawn from two independent sources A and B. We can cross-classify the patients by source as in Table 14.9. The two sources are analogous to the two sets of traps. Since the two sources are assumed independent, the odds ratio must be 1, that is, ad = bc, so the best estimate for d (the 'missing' individuals not discovered by either method) is:

$$d = \frac{bc}{a}$$

In practice, it is best to have several sources for identifying subjects and the statistical method used is log-linear modelling. This is rather like multiple regression where the predictor variables are ones or zeroes, depending on whether the subject was detected by that source or not, and the outcome vari-able is the predicted count of individuals. The sources do not have to be inde-pendent as this can be allowed for by extra predictor variables denoting interactions between sources. The estimate of the number missing is then obtained by extrapolation to the situation in which all the predictor variables are zero. Assumptions are:
- that the population is closed (i.e. no migration in or out during the interval covered by the study)
- consistent methods for defining cases of the condition
- no errors in classifying subjects

Table 14.9 Basic layout for capture–recapture		
Source A	Source B	
	Found	Not Found
Found	a	b
Not Found	c	d = ?

- each subject must be ascertainable in principle from at least two sources (though the probabilities of this may vary from source to source).

An example is the paper by Smeeton et al.[17]

Disease clusters

Cancer registries and public health departments are often approached by individuals with concerns on the lines that 'there seems to be an awful lot of cancer cases lately in this area'. Points to bear in mind are that cancer is not one disease and 'common cancers occur commonly', especially as a population grows older. Moreover, not only is the 'incubation period' for cancers measurable in decades but it is also variable, so that the causes of cancers now occurring, usually lie in the distant past and have little to do with present circumstances (especially as people will have moved into and out of the area over this time).

In the past, evidence for clustering in both space and time has been sought as evidence for contagion, notably in classic studies of childhood leukaemia and Burkitt's lymphoma.[18,19] However, space–time clustering can be caused by factors other than case-to-case transmission; possibilities are migration of susceptible populations, uneven adoption over time of diagnostic facilities or fashions, or spread of an aetiological agent (not necessarily infectious) from a wandering source.[20] For these reasons and the fact that even diseases known to be infectious may give equivocal or negative results, interest has since rather declined.[21] A useful, if now old, review of methods to detect space–time clustering was given by Smith[22] but, significantly perhaps, an updated version of that chapter was not included in subsequent editions.

Generally it is most likely that investigation of disease clusters (including space–time clustering) will be most fruitful when the disease has a short incubation period and most cases are overtly diseased. In addition, it is helpful if a suspected point source of exposure exists; for example, in the studies by Bhopal[23,24] on legionnaire's disease. With regard to cancers, virtually all allegations of a cluster turn out to be no excess at all; of the remainder, few result in demonstration of a cause. In cancer, therefore, what is most likely to be a real 'signal' and worth investigating is when multiple cases of a single uncommon type occur, when many cases are seen in children or when there is a common occupational link. However, even then there is an awkward question to be answered, if a real cluster is established, what if anything will or even can be done about it?

When there is a suspected point source or occupational risk the problem is best resolved by standard case–control or cohort approaches. Practical advice is given in the handbook published by the Leukaemia Research Fund.[25]

The need to allow for spatial correlation

When we compare, for instance, cancer incidence rates or between different geographical areas or survival rates between different hospital trusts, it is tempting to treat each area or trust as if they were independent. Thinking realistically, this is not very likely if the areas are adjacent (for example, local authorities) or have overlapping catchment populations. The correlation between such areas or institutions is likely to decline the further apart they are, and the phenomenon is termed spatial autocorrelation. The effect is to distort the standard errors that are obtained using standard methods. The solution is to use more sophisticated methods which allow for the presence of the autocorrelation, but which are more familiar to geographers than to the medical community. Special advice should be sought but some of the technicalities of the topic have been reviewed, for a medical rather than a geographical audience, by Pickle.[26]

Time series

Time series consist of observations over time; for example the number of daily admissions to a maternity unit. There are various analyses that can be helpful for epidemiological purposes. Appropriate tests exist to detect (or confirm) the presence of seasonality in admissions for a particular cause, although these tests are less likely to be performed if software for Poisson or logistic regression is available.[27,28] Matsuda[29] provides an example, which also includes the raw data.

Other time series applications include the monitoring of clinical performance and evaluation of disease incidence 'before' and 'after' some intervention.[30,31] Specialised routines are needed to allow for the autocorrelation seen in such data (observations close in time are more likely to be related than those far apart). The problem is related to that in spatial analysis but is simpler, so that appropriate software is easier to find.

Age–period–cohort models use large data sets (typically population-based mortality or cancer incidence data) collected over many year to disentangle the influences of age, period of death (secular trend) and cohort (generation) on disease incidence or mortality rates, using Poisson regression. This can be a difficult task because of the non-identifiability problem: if any two of the three variables are known, the third (for which only non-linear effects can be estimated) is determined exactly. There are various approaches to handling the problem.

Conclusion

The key areas addressed by epidemiology are aetiology, diagnosis and prognosis. These broad concepts can be applied to and illuminate all branches of medicine; in a sense, epidemiology can be regarded as the true theoretical basis of all medicine, because its concerns are not constrained by accidents of physiology.

References
1. Gardner M, Donnan S. Life expectancy: variations among regional health authorities. *Popul Trends* 1977;10:10–12.
2. Purdie E, editor. *Guide to Official Statistics*. Office for National Statistics. London: HMSO; 1996.

3. Hill AB. The clinical trial. *N Engl J Med* 1952;247:113–19.
4. Wignall BK, Fox AJ. Mortality of female gas mask assemblers. *Br J Ind Med* 1982;39:34–8.
5. Barker D. The midwife, the coincidence, and the hypothesis. *BMJ* 2003;327:1428–30.
6. Doll R, Hill AB. A study of the aetiology of carcinoma of the lung. *Br Med J* 1952;2:1271–86.
7. Hammond EC, Horn D. Smoking and death rates – report on forty-four months of follow-up of 187,783 men. *J Am Med Assoc* 1958;166:1294–308.
8. Suissa S. The case-time-control design. *Epidemiology* 1995;3:248–53.
9. Maclure M. The case-crossover design: a method for studying transient effects on the risk of acute events. *Am J Epidemiol* 1991 ;1332:144–53.
10. Walker AM, Jick H, Hunter JR, Danford A, Watkins RN, Alhadeff L, *et al.* Vasectomy and non-fatal myocardial infarction. *Lancet* 1981;i(8210):13–15.
11. Farrington CP, Nash J, Miller E. Case series analysis of adverse reactions to vaccines: a comparative evaluation. *Am J Epidemiol* 1996;143:1165–73. Erratum in: *Am J Epidemiol* 1998;147:93.
12. Cummings P, McKnight B, Greenland S. Matched cohort methods for injury research. *Epidemiol Rev* 2003;25:43–50.
13. Sackett DL, Haynes RB, Guyatt GH, Tugwell P. *Clinical Epidemiology: A Basic Science for Clinical Medicine*. 2nd ed. Boston: Little Brown and Company; 1991.
14. Lambourne A, Lederer H. Effects of observer variation in population screening for cervical carcinoma. *J Clin Pathol* 1973;26:564–9.
15. Landis JR, Koch GG. The measurement of observer agreement for categorical criteria. *Biometrics* 1977;33,159–74.
16. Theodossi A, Skene AM, Portmann B, Knill-Jones RP, Patrick RS, Tate RA, *et al.* Observer variation in assessment of liver biopsies including analysis by kappa statistics. *Gastroenterology* 1980;79,232–41.
17. Smeeton NC, Rona RJ, Sharland G, Botting BJ, Barnett A, Dundas R. Estimating the prevalence of malformation of the heart in the first year of life using capture-recapture methods. *Am J Epidemiol* 1999;150:778–85.
18. Knox G. Epidemiology of childhood leukaemia in Northumberland and Durham. *Brit J Prev Soc Med* 1964;18:17–24.
19. Pike MC, Williams EH, Wright B. Burkitt's tumour in the West Nile District of Uganda 1961–65. *Br Med J* 1967;2:395–9.
20. Doll R. *Prevention of Cancer. Pointers from Epidemiology*. London: Nuffield Provincial Hospitals Trust; 1967.
21. Goldacre MJ. Space-time and family characteristics of meningococcal disease and hemophilus meningitis. *Int J Epidemiol* 1977;6:101–5.
22. Smith PG. Spatial and temporal clustering. In: Schottenfeld D, Fraumeni JF, editors. *Cancer Epidemiology and Prevention*. Philadelphia, PA: Saunders; 1982. p. 391–407.
23. Bhopal RS, Fallon RJ, Buist EC, Black RJ, Urquhart JD. Proximity of the home to a cooling tower and risk of non-outbreak Legionnaires' disease. *BMJ* 1991;302:378–83.
24. Bhopal RS, Diggle P, Rowlingson B. Pinpointing clusters of apparently sporadic cases of Legionnaires' disease. *BMJ* 1992;304:1022–7.

25. Arrundale J, Bain M, Botting B, Brewster D, Cartwright R, Chalmers J, *et al.* *Handbook and Guide to the Investigation of Clusters of Diseases.* Leeds: Leukaemia Research Fund; 1997.

26. Pickle LW. Spatial analysis of disease. *Cancer Treat Res.* 2002;113:113–50.

27. Edwards JH. The recognition and estimation of cyclic trends. *Ann Hum Genetic* 1961;25:83–7.

28. Walter SD, Elwood JM. A test for seasonality of events with a variable population at risk. *Br J Prev Soc Med* 1975;29:18–21.

29. Matsuda S and Kahyo H. Seasonality of preterm births in Japan. *Int J Epidemiol* 1992;21:91–100.

30. Catalano R, Serxner S. Time series designs of potential interest to epidemiologists. *Am J Epidemiol.* 1987;126;724–31.

31. Helfenstein U. The use of transfer function models, intervention analysis and related time series methods in epidemiology. *Int J Epidemiol* 1991;20:808–15.

32. Rodrigues L, Kirkwood BR. Case–control designs in the study of common diseases: updates on the demise of the rare disease assumption and the choice of sampling scheme for controls. *Int J Epidemiol* 1990;19:205–13.

Further reading

Basic

dos Santos Silva I. *Cancer Epidemiology: principles and methods.* Lyon: International Agency for Research on Cancer; 1999.

Fletcher RH, Fletcher SW, Wagner EH. *Clinical Epidemiology. The essentials.* 3rd ed. Baltimore: Williams and Wilkins; 1996.

Friedman GD. *Primer of Epidemiology.* 3rd ed. New York: McGraw Hill; 1994.

Kahn HA, Sempos CT. *Statistical Methods in Epidemiology.* Oxford: Oxford University Press; 1989.

Lilienfeld DE, Stolley PD. *Foundations of Epidemiology.* 3rd ed. Oxford: Oxford University Press; 1994.

MacMahon B, Trichopulos D. *Epidemiology. Principles and Methods.* 2nd ed. Boston: Little Brown; 1996.

Stolley PD, Lasky T. *Investigating Disease Patterns. The Science of Epidemiology.* Scientific American Library. New York: WH Freeman; 1995.

Advanced

Breslow NE, Day NE. *Statistical Methods in Cancer Research I. The Analysis of Case–Control Studies.* Lyon: International Agency for research on Cancer; 1980.

Breslow NE, Day NE. *Statistical Methods in Cancer Research II. The Design and Analysis of Cohort Studies.* Lyon: International Agency for Research on Cancer; 1987.

Esteve J, Benhamou E, Raymond L. *Statistical Methods in Cancer Research IV. Descriptive Epidemiology.* Lyon: International Agency for Research on Cancer; 1994.

Mahesh K, Parmar B, Machin D. *Survival Analysis. A Practical Approach.* Chichester: John Wiley; 1995.

Morrison AS. *Screening in Chronic Disease.* Oxford: Oxford University Press; 1985.

15

Ethics, ethics committees, consent and fraud

Richard Kerr-Wilson

'So act as to treat humanity, whether in thine own person or in that of
another, in every case as an end withal, never as means only.'

(Immanuel Kant 1724–1804)[1]

In the short time since the publication of the first edition of this book, ethics
in research and research ethics committees have changed significantly. New
challenges have evolved with the expansion of science, such as the mapping of
the human genome and the development of stem cell research. The need for
ethical review of research has become more accepted by researchers and the
process by which this is carried out more structured. Increasing public awareness has resulted in more stringent requirements for consent and proposals
for legislation. On the negative side, increasing commercial pressure has
meant that fraud has expanded from the individual case to the corporate.

Ethics and research

Ethics can variously be defined as 'rules of conduct', 'the science of morals',
'the science of human duty' or 'the practical application of right and wrong'.
In science, scientific method requires testing of a hypothesis against observed
facts. For research in science to be ethical, the hypothesis should be reasonable, carried out honestly, with a good chance of both being completed and
answering the question posed, and should carry the minimum of risks. Similar
criteria can be applied to medical research: benefits must outweigh risks;
results should not be fabricated and should be disclosed honestly and openly.
The research does not always have to be testing a new idea; sometimes,
research is required to confirm or refute earlier investigations or translate previous research to different populations. In addition, in medical research, as far
as possible, the subject of the research should understand and agree to the
aims of the research, and appreciate the benefits and risks involved.

Most people would agree that some form of external ethical review in
medical research is necessary.[2] Researchers may be too close to their subject
or conscious of demands from other directions to appreciate the wider implications of their work. If the research is sponsored they may be under financial
constraints to produce data or withhold results. Likewise, academic pressure
may cause them to manipulate or fabricate their findings. Researchers themselves may consider ethical review to be an irksome, even pointless, hurdle to

be jumped before they can begin their work. Nevertheless, it is advisable to give some thought to the ethical issues in the early stages of discussing a research proposal. This will help to ensure that the research is appropriate and relevant. It will save time and improve the chances of the research being completed and the results accepted. Ethics has to be part of scientific enquiry and conduct, not a separate field.[3]

Ethics in medical research are an example of situational ethics, meaning that the process is dynamic and not absolute.[4] Research ethics are related in both time and place to the surrounding culture. For example, James Marion Sims' work on vesicovaginal fistula was acceptable in 19th century Alabama but may not be considered so today.[5] Even now, there is controversy as to whether research projects linking affluent universities in economically developed countries with slums and villages of the developing world are appropriate. It is questionable whether truly ethical research is possible across such a gradient. Following a case–control study of HIV-1 in Haiti, 15 participants were asked to take an oral examination on the contents of the consent form; only three passed.[6] The Declaration of Helsinki on the ethical principles for medical research involving human subjects states in paragraph 30: 'At the conclusion of the study, every patient entered into the study should be assured of access to the best proven prophylactic, diagnostic and therapeutic methods identified by the study'.[7] It would be interesting research in itself to find out how often this was applied, particularly to research carried out in developing countries.

The need for ethical review in medical research is relatively recent. Even 25 years ago it was not considered obligatory. The increased requirement has come about partly as a result of more emphasis on individual autonomy and choice but also from increased media interest and public perception, greater scientific knowledge of adverse effects and advances in science itself. Individual choice and autonomy have succeeded the professional paternalism of Sims' day. Subjects expect to be asked if they would like to participate in a research project, to be informed of the advantages and disadvantages and even of the results. Adverse effects may not be apparent for many years to come; a radiological study of the bladder during labour was acceptable 50 years ago but would not be considered ethical today. New techniques, such as cloning of embryos, stem cell research and the mapping of the human genome, present questions that have not arisen before and may affect the whole population, not just the individual.

Ethical analysis of research

Ethical analysis of research can be approached in three different ways: goal-based, duty-based and rights-based.[8] The goal-based researcher will consider that ends justify means, that what is achieved for the benefit of mankind as a result of the research justifies the way in which that research is carried out. The outcome is all-important. This would be the justification made by doctors carrying out experiments on prisoners or concentration camp inmates; it is the antithesis of Kant's philosophy. Pure goal-based research is generally considered to be repugnant and most researchers will acknowledge that they have a duty-based responsibility to their research subjects to cause them minimum harm.

The third, rights-based approach considers the research subject first and asks whether the subject is satisfied with the purpose and method of the research. This requires adequate information to be provided and consent obtained.

Medical research should be a balance between these three approaches; if one aspect is emphasised to the detriment of the others, research will be compromised. Each case will be different and the weighting given to each approach will be different. It is the job of the research ethics committee to establish this balance when evaluating a research proposal.

Published guidelines

Many national and international bodies have issued statements on biomedical research involving human subjects. The World Medical Assembly adopted the original Declaration of Helsinki in 1964. This is entitled: 'Ethical Principles for Medical Research Involving Human Subjects' and was last amended in Edinburgh in 2000, with a note of clarification in Washington in 2002.[7] Although this is not a legal requirement, it provides an internationally recognised ethical standard. All biomedical research should be conducted according to the recommendations it contains. Paragraph 13 states that an experimental protocol: 'should be submitted for consideration, comment, guidance, and where appropriate, approval to a specially appointed ethical review committee, which must be independent of the investigator, the sponsor or any other kind of undue influence ... The committee has the right to monitor continuing trials'. Paragraph 16: 'The design of all studies should be publicly available'.

Under paragraph 27, it states: 'Negative as well as positive results should be published or otherwise publicly available ... Reports of experimentation not in accordance with the principles laid down in this Declaration should not be accepted for publication'.

The Convention on Human Rights and Biomedicine of the Council of Europe, adopted in 1997,[9] states under article 16 that research on a person may only be undertaken if:

- there is no alternative
- the risks incurred are not disproportionate to the benefits
- the research project has been approved by the competent body
- the persons undergoing research have been informed of their rights
- the necessary consent has been given and is documented.

In February 2002, the General Medical Council (GMC) in the UK, published guidance on *Research: the role and responsibilities of doctors*.[10] This guidance discusses the definition of research, as well as the principles governing research and putting the principles into practice. It states that:

- research projects must be completed, unless results indicate that patients may be harmed or no benefit can be expected
- records and reports must be kept accurately
- patients must not be pressurised to participate
- if patients are being put at risk or there is evidence of fraud, this must be reported
- conflicts of interest must be declared.

The role of ethics committees

All medical research involving human subjects should be reviewed by a research ethics committee (REC), whether it is being undertaken in hospital, a primary care facility, a research laboratory or the community. Sometimes, it can be difficult to know whether a project is research and should be submitted to an ethics committee or is part of an audit. The GMC defines medical research as 'any experimental study into the causes, treatment or prevention of ill health and disease in humans, involving people or their tissues or organs or data'.[10] It includes epidemiological research, including analysis of medical records and whether anonymised. It does not include audit, which involves no experimental study. In theory, audit is retrospective, comparing practice to a standard, whereas research is prospective, testing a hypothesis. In practice, this distinction is not always clear. One audit office has offered the following yardstick: if you can answer 'yes' to the first of the two following questions and 'no' to the third, then it is probably audit; if not, it is probably research:

1. Is the purpose of the proposed project to try to improve the quality of patient care in the local setting?
2. Will the project involve measuring practice against standards?
3. Does the project involve anything being done to patients which would not have been part of their routine management?[11]

The purpose of RECs is to encourage good research, not to obstruct or discourage it. They should weigh the benefits of the research against the risks to the subjects, protect participants from undue harm and discourage fraud and unsatisfactory results. They should review research design, making sure that the aim of the research is reasonable and the methods proposed are likely to provide an answer to the question posed. They should ensure that suitably qualified personnel will carry out the research, following an appropriate protocol. The number of subjects required to provide a valid conclusion must be reasonable and it must be possible to recruit them within the time suggested. Appropriate technological backup and statistical support should be available, with the necessary funds to support this. Subjects should be informed that they are involved in a research project; given details of it and allowed to withdraw at any time without detriment to their care.[7] Their consent to participate should be freely given whenever possible, and documented. They should be advised what will happen when the research is finished, both to them and to the results. Ethics committees themselves should keep a register of research proposals, and make sure all results of research are made publicly available. RECs are not constituted to review more general ethical problems, which should be referred to a more appropriate body.

Operational procedures

New operating procedures in the UK came into use on 1 March 2004.[12] This was in response to Directive 2001/20/EC of the European Parliament,[13] which was implemented by statutory regulations in the UK on 1 May 2004. The European Union (EU) directive was set up to facilitate commercial drug development and to give Europe a competitive edge in the pharmaceuticals market. It provides protection for vulnerable patients such as children (under the age of 16 years) and incapacitated adults but at the same time specifies mandatory inspection of trial sites and the threat of enforcement. Although the European Union Directive applies to all clinical trials on human subjects involving medicinal products, the UK procedures go further. They cover all research ethics committees in the UK and all applications for review of any health-related research.

Operating procedures for research ethics committees are beset by acronyms. All research committees, which review proposals, which come under the EU Directive must be recognised by the UK Ethics Committee Authority (UKECA). Local RECs (LRECs) still exist but there is now a Central Office for RECs (COREC), which coordinates the work of all research ethics committees and provides advice, support and monitoring. All ethics committees in the UK should operate under the new operating procedures, some of which have superseded the previously published Governance Arrangements for Research Ethics Committees (GaFREC).[14]

The new procedures mean a more centralised system with deadlines for the research to be approved and a single generic application form. All applications for ethical review are assessed by one REC only. A decision by the committee on a valid research proposal must be made within 60 days. This decision then becomes binding for all the UK.

All RECs meet monthly. All research proposals, apart from single-site research not involving a medicinal product, must go through the Central Allocation System and be reviewed by a main REC. Single site research not involving a medicinal product can be reviewed by the local committee.

An REC should consist of 12–18 members with balanced age and gender distribution. They should include a mixture of experts and at least three lay members. Whenever possible, members from ethnic backgrounds and people with disabilities should be included. Members can serve for no more than two terms of 3–5 years. A quorum of seven members is stipulated, which must include the chairman or vice-chairman, one expert member and one lay member. Independent decisions by the chairman are no longer allowed.[12,14] Members should declare any conflicts of interest and withdraw from the discussion if this occurs. If a member of a committee is also a named researcher, the application should be submitted to another REC.

When a research proposal is ready for submission by the chief investigator with overall responsibility for the research, the COREC application form should be completed before contacting the office of the Central Allocation System. The main REC will then be allocated and a reference number given. The number must be entered on the form, parts A and B of which must be submitted to the main REC, preferably electronically, within 4 days of booking. Supporting documentation, such as the patient information sheet and the consent form, should accompany the application form. A letter confirming validation will be sent to the chief investigator within 5 days.

It is important that research proposals for ethical review are fully prepared before submission, since the 60-day clock starts ticking on the date the REC receives a valid application. The REC can only request clarification on specific issues once before a decision is made. If the response is considered unsatisfactory by the REC, the proposal may be rejected.

If the research is multi-site, once the chief investigator receives the letter from the main REC confirming the application to be valid, the principal investigator at each site can be instructed to apply for site-specific assessment, usually to the local REC. This consists of part C of the standard REC application form, giving a summary of the proposal, together with the CV of the principal investigator only. The site-specific assessment assesses the suitability of the local investigator and the local arrangements but cannot change any of the protocol, the consent form or the information sheet. The site-specific assessor notifies the main REC of their decision within 25 days; after this time, a reminder is sent to ensure the overall time limit of 60 days is adhered to. Additional sites can be added at a later stage by the same process. Applicants are advised of the ethical opinion of the main REC within 60 days.

Research should normally commence within 12 months of the date on which a favourable ethical opinion is given by an REC. A study is generally considered to have commenced when the first subject gives written informed consent to participate.[12]

Progress reports should be submitted to the main REC at least annually. A clinical trial is said to have been concluded when the last patient has had their last visit. The ethics committee should be notified that a clinical trial has ended within 90 days.[13]

Any substantial amendments to the protocol that affect patient safety or the conduct of the trial and occur after the trial has started, such as a change in informed consent or recruitment procedures, should be submitted to the main REC for review. Their decision should be given within 35 days.

These operating procedures are still relatively new but it is hoped that they will avoid some of the delay and duplication that not infrequently occurred during the process of ethical review in the past.

Informed consent

The EU Directive[13] states that informed consent is a 'decision, which must be written, dated and signed, to take part in a clinical trial, taken freely after being duly informed of its nature, significance, implications and risks and appropriately documented, by any person capable of giving consent, or, where the person is not capable of giving consent, by his or her legal representative'. The idea of consent is not new but the doctrine of informed consent is relatively recent, an early example being cited in a tale of mesmerism by Edgar Allan Poe.[15] The concept of informed consent is a result of the shift in attitude from paternalistic concern by the researcher for his subject to the self-determination and autonomy of the volunteers themselves.[16]

Although usually considered as a whole, informed consent consists of three parts: the voluntary agreement of the participant, which is not new, the more recent duty to disclose sufficient information before agreement is reached[17] and the comprehension of this information. Fully informed consent is an unattainable ideal, since a description of what may occur can never be exhaustive. A complete list of circumstances that may arise during a particular piece of research is not feasible. Not only is complete disclosure impossible but there is also a question of the degree of comprehension that is required. A decision not to participate in research may be made from ignorance; likewise, agreement to take part may also be based on poor comprehension. The example of the lack of understanding of the consent form in a study of HIV-1 transmission in Haiti has already been mentioned.[6] Comprehension and informed consent were also assessed in a study on myocardial infarction; the patient information sheet was written at an educational level for 18-year-olds; only 18% read the information sheet before giving or refusing consent, and 18% were not considered competent to consent.[18] Admittedly, this was a trial undertaken in a clinical emergency but without such objective assessment an individual's comprehension may be difficult to assess. Consent is probably more important than obsessive pursuit of the unattainable Holy Grail of providing total information and requiring full comprehension.

Perhaps of more importance in practical terms is that the consent is genuine.[19] Effective communication is the key; information should be provided in terms and in a form that can be understood.[10] Researchers should communicate the purpose of the research and its expected benefits, the procedures and risks involved and the option to withdraw without penalty at any time. Individuals should be informed that ethics committee approval has been obtained. If randomisation is involved, the reasons for it and the process should be explained. Participants must be told who will have access to the records. It should be clear what information will be available at the end of the research, where this will be available and the likely duration of the research. Details of compensation in the event of injury should be made clear. The information should be provided in written form in a language that is comprehensible to patients, volunteers or relatives.

A third party, such as a research nurse, is probably the best person to provide the information, in order to avoid bias or undue pressure by the researcher. There should be time to assimilate the information and to discuss it with others if requested. An opportunity should be given to talk with the nurse or researcher before asking the volunteer to sign that they have read and understood the information and agree to participate in the research. If all reasonable care is exercised, adequate and genuine consent may be established, even though it can never be 'fully informed'.

Special considerations

Legal capacity to consent requires an individual to be able to receive information, understand it and act upon it. The EU Directive[13] states that people who are incapable of giving legal consent should be given special protection. It specifically mentions children and psychiatric patients. The GMC (definition)[10] includes frail elderly people, people living in institutions and adults with learning difficulties, as well as pregnant women and children. Pregnant women may be consenting for their unborn child as well as themselves, at a time when they are particularly vulnerable.[20] Other areas for special consideration are research in emergencies and the use of retained tissue for subsequent research.

Vulnerable individuals in the categories mentioned should not be excluded from research which may be of significant benefit to them but should not be included if the same results can be obtained by using people who are competent to give their consent. Normally, they should only be included in clinical trials if the research has the potential to produce real and direct benefit to the individual's health. Their participation should be limited to areas of research related to their incapacity. If they are incapable of giving informed consent themselves, then written consent should be obtained from their legal representative. This may be either a lay person, selected by virtue of their relationship with the person concerned, such as a spouse; or a professional legal representative, such as a solicitor or doctor, if no one is able to act as a personal legal representative. Consent must represent the subject's presumed will and can be withdrawn. If the person lacking capacity has previously indicated preferences by means of an advance statement or directive, this must be respected. The person not able to give consent must receive information according to his or her level of understanding, which can, if necessary, include such material as drawings.

Non-therapeutic research, which is not intended to benefit the individual directly, may be carried out on patients who lack mental capacity, as long as it is into the condition from which the patient suffers and will not expose the participant to more than negligible risk.[21]

The problem of obtaining consent to research in emergencies has been recognised by the Food and Drug Administration in the USA.[22] Research on human subjects in need of emergency intervention but who cannot give consent because of their medical condition, is permitted provided the subject is in a life-threatening situation and available treatments are unproven or unsatisfactory. The proposal must be approved by the institutional review board and the risks associated with the procedure must be reasonable. The subject or their representative must be informed as soon as possible of their inclusion in the study, and their option to withdraw.

Research on women in labour has in the past been permitted by ethics committees without insisting on informed consent, because of the difficulty in obtaining this intrapartum.[23] However, it is recommended that if such research is contemplated, information should be provided beforehand, such as in the antenatal clinic, to provide adequate time for explanation and discussion. Women will then be in a better position to give consent, which should be requested at the time of randomisation or treatment.[20]

The problem of research on human tissue is the subject of the Human Tissue Act 2004. The legislation arose as a result of the public outcry that arose after the discovery that organs of dead children had been removed and stored for unspecified future research without proper consent. The initial drafts of the Bill provoked strong criticism, particularly in the areas of anonymity, generic consent and the composition of the Human Tissue Authority.[24] If human tissue is removed at surgery, appropriate consent must be obtained for the retention of the tissue for research and further specific consent for any subsequent research project.

Further details about the practicalities of obtaining informed consent are included in Chapter 16.

Fraud

Scientific fraud can be defined as any deliberate attempt to mislead during the application or performance of research or its publication. Fraud is not just sloppy research but intentional misconduct.[25] It involves deliberate deception and may take the form of fabricating or withholding data or even inventing patients who do not exist. Forgery of approval by an ethics committee may occur to allow research to take place[26] or data manipulated to provide the desired answer.

No one knows the extent of fraud in research, since it is probably only the most blatant cases that are detected. Few cases appeared until the 1980s; in the USA, only 12 cases of scientific misconduct were disclosed between 1974 and 1981, and in Britain, only five had been documented by the end of 1988.[26,27] Since then, numbers seem to have escalated. In the USA, the Office of Research Integrity was set up in 1992 and 10 years later, the 2002 Annual Report mentioned 191 allegations made, 41 new cases opened and 13 of 32 cases closed that year which involved falsification and/or fabrication.[28]

Fraud may be individual or, increasingly, corporate. The motive for individual fraud may be to enhance academic reputation, for financial gain, as a result of psychiatric illness or merely vanity.[27] The pressure to 'publish or perish' in academic institutions, with academic excellence measured in numbers of publications, must make fraud increasingly tempting. Significant fees are paid for enrolling patients into trials by commercial companies, with the result that occasionally nonexistent patients have been entered for the researcher to receive payment. Alternatively, names of real patients may have been used, without the patients actually being enrolled in the study.[29] Two of the more notorious cases in the past were the report in 1994 of the successful relocation of an ectopic pregnancy, when the patient never existed, and the forging of consent forms for patients who never received the drug on trial. In both cases, the doctors concerned were in senior positions in their profession and working in teaching hospitals.[30]

In current times, with increasing commercialisation of research, fraud has spread to the corporate world. This has become particularly apparent in the under-reporting of results, the failure to publish negative results or concealing results that may be detrimental to the marketing of a product. Less than one-third of 158 clinical trials approved by one ethics committee had been published 3 years after completion and only 27% of trials that had been started had been presented at a scientific meeting. Eleven trials had not even started.[31] Although it is highly unlikely that the other trials were deliberate fraud, they nevertheless misled those who had taken part voluntarily, in the belief that the trial would be completed and the results made public.

The problem of unpublished data has lately been exemplified in the use of paroxetine for depressed children. Although published data suggested a favourable risk–benefit profile, unpublished data indicated that risks could outweigh benefits to treat depression in children and young people, with an increase in suicidal behaviour.[32] The suggestion has been made that the unfavourable results were deliberately withheld to promote the marketing of the product. A lawsuit has been filed against the manufacturer, accusing them of fraud and seeking return of all profits obtained through fraudulent means.[33]

A more sinister example of commercial pressure to prevent publication of adverse results is that involving the drug deferiprone, which was being tested at the Hospital for Sick Children in Toronto for the treatment of thalassaemia major. When it was found that the drug was not only ineffective but might actually be toxic, the Research Ethics Board was advised and the researcher was recommended to inform other physicians and the appropriate authorities. The manufacturer terminated the trial and threatened legal action if any of the information was divulged to others.[34]

The detection and prevention of fraud is not easy. Individual fraud is less likely to occur when the researcher is junior and is still under supervision. It is more difficult to detect when the researcher is at a senior level in his or her career and is no longer supervised. Corporate fraud may be even more difficult to discover, because of financial pressures and vested interests. No single measure will eliminate fraud but methods to decrease the occurrence can be taken by the REC, by the participants themselves and by the editors of journals.

Ethics committees should require registration of all research proposals submitted to them. They should request an annual progress report[12] as well as final results, with information on how these will be made publicly available.[8] Since 1 May 2004, all interventional clinical trials of medicinal products in the EU must also be entered on a European database (EudraCT). Although it is not a statutory requirement, ethics committees could also help to eliminate fraud by carrying out random audits of protocols submitted. When a proposal is referred for ethical review, researchers are advised that subjects may be contacted in order to audit ethical aspects of the research and asked to identify patients for this purpose. A simple questionnaire is then sent to a selected number of patients to verify that they understand and have consented to participate in the research project.[35] This process will help to eliminate bogus research subjects, although it will not prevent the fabrication and manipulation of data.

Volunteers participating in research can also help to eliminate fraud. They should insist on publicly accessible information about the trial and that the investigators undertake to make the results publicly available within a reasonable time after its conclusion. If these conditions are not met, they should withhold their consent.[36]

To further ensure that all trials are in the public domain and avoid selective reporting, the International Committee of Medical Journal Editors stated, in 2004, that all member journals will require, as a condition of consideration for publication, trials to be registered in a public registry before the start of patient enrolment.[37] No specific registry is specified, but several criteria must be met. Journal editors could go further by including in their instructions to authors advice that random requests to review raw data may be made. Researchers would have to ensure that data were kept in a retrievable form and submitted if requested. Such a procedure would go some way towards preventing the forging of data and help make research both accurate and ethical.

Conclusions

In the last few years there have been major changes in the conduct of ethical review of clinical research in the UK and Europe. Ethical review is now an accepted part of the research procedure and has become more unified and better organised. At the same time, fraud has become apparent on a larger scale. It is hoped that some of the measures proposed and put in place will make research more transparent and results more publicly available.

Useful websites
Central Office for Research Ethics Committees: www.corec.org.uk
Declaration of Helsinki: www.wma.net/e/policy/b3.htm

References

1. Kant I. *Fundamental Principles of the Metaphysic of Morals 1785. The Critique of Practical Reason.* 6th ed. Thomas Kinsmill Abbot, translator. London: Longmans Green; 1963.
2. Kerr-Wilson R. Problems with the ethics of medical research. *Br J Hosp Med* 1994;52:495–6.
3. Fylkesnes K, Fylkesnes TK. Informed consent as part and parcel of the scientific enquiry. *Lancet* 2003;361:2171–2.
4. Cefalo RC, Berghmans RL, Hall SP. The bioethics of human fetal tissue research and therapy: moral decision making of professionals. *Am J Obstet Gynecol* 1994;170:12–19.
5. Ojanuga D. The medical ethics of the 'father of gynaecology', Dr J Marion Sims. *J Med Ethics* 1993;19:28–31.
6. Fitzgerald DW, Marotte C, Verdier RI, Johnson WD, Pape JW. Comprehension during informed consent in a less-developed country. *Lancet* 2002;360:1301–2.
7. World Medical Association Declaration of Helsinki. Ethical Principles for Medical Research Involving Human Subjects. World Medical Assembly. *J Postgrad Med* 2002;48:206–8.
8. Foster C. Teaching members of research ethics committees: systematic ethical analysis and virtue ethics. *King's College, London: Dispatches* 1997;7:1–2.
9. Council of Europe. 1996 Convention on Human Rights and Biomedicine. *Bull Med Ethics* 1997;125:13–19.
10. General Medical Council. *Research: The Role and Responsibility of Doctors.* London: General Medical Council; 2002.
11. University of Bristol Healthcare Trust Clinical Audit Central Office. *How to Tell the Difference Between Audit and Research.* Bristol: UBHT; 2000.
12. Central Office for Research and Ethics Committees. *Standard Operating Procedures for Research Ethics Committees in the United Kingdom.* Version 1.0. London: NHS; 2004.
13. Directive 2001/20/EC of the European Parliament and of the Council of 4 April 2001 on the approximation of the law and administrative provisions of the Member States relating to the implementation of good clinical practice in the conduct of clinical trials on medicinal products for human use. *Official Journal of the European Communities* 2001;L121/34–44.
14. Department of Health. *Governance Arrangements for Research Ethics Committees.* London: Department of Health; 2001.
15. Altschuler EL. Informed consent in an Edgar Allan Poe tale. *Lancet* 2003;362:1504.
16. Templeton A. Informed consent. In: Bewley S and Ward RH, editors. *Ethics in Obstetrics and Gynaecology.* London: RCOG Press; 1994. p. 287–97.
17. Sreenivasan G. Does informed consent to research require comprehension? *Lancet* 2003;362:2016–8.

18. Williams BF, French JK, White HD. Informed consent during the clinical emergency of acute myocardial infarction (HERO-2 consent substudy): a prospective observational study. *Lancet* 2003;361:918–22.
19. Nuffield Council on Bioethics. *Human Tissue: Ethical and Legal Issues.* London: Nuffield Council on Bioethics; 1995. p. 44–5.
20. AIMS, the National Childbirth Trust and the Maternity Alliance. A charter for ethical research in maternity care. *Bull Med Ethics* 1997;130:8–11.
21. Lord Chancellor's Department. *Who decides? Making Decisions on Behalf of Mentally Incapacitated Adults.* London: HMSO; 1997.
22. Food and Drug Administration. Protection of human subjects: informed consent. *Bull Med Ethics* 1997;132:9–11.
23. Westgren M, Kruger K, Ek S, Grunevald C, Kublickas M, Naka K, *et al.* Lactate compared with pH analysis at fetal scalp blood sampling: a prospective randomised study. *Br J Obstet Gynaecol* 1998;105:29–33.
24. Pincock S. The law of consent. *Lancet* 2004;364:489–90.
25. Kansu E, Ruacan S. Research ethics and scientific misconduct in biomedical research. *Acta Neurochir Suppl* 2002;83:11–15.
26. Wells F, Blunt J. The role of LRECs in the prevention of fraud. *Bull Med Ethics* 1997;131:2.
27. Royal College of Physicians. *Fraud and Misconduct in Medical Research. Causes, Investigation and Prevention.* London: Royal College of Physicians; 1991.
28. Office of Research Integrity [http://ori.dhhs.gov/international/activity/index.shtml].
29. Hoeksma HL, Troost J, Grobbee DE, Wiersinga WM, van Wijmen FC, Klasen EC. A case of fraud in a neurological pharmaceutical clinical trial. *Ned Tijdschr Geneeskd* 2003;147:1372–7.
30. Mihill C. Falsified research 'threat to patients'. *The Guardian* 1997; 6 November.
31. Pich J, Carné X, Arnaiz J-A, Gómez B, Trilla A, Rodés J. Role of a research ethics committee in follow-up and publication of results. *Lancet* 2003;361:1015–16.
32. Whittington CJ, Kendall T, Fonagy P, Cottrell D, Cotgrove D, Boddington E. Selective serotonin reuptake inhibitors in childhood depression: systematic review of published versus unpublished data. *Lancet* 2004;363:1341–5.
33. Editorial. Is GSK guilty of fraud? *Lancet* 2004;363:1919.
34. Baylis F. The Olivieri debacle: where were the heroes of bioethics? *J Med Ethics* 2004;30:44–9.
35. Berry J. Local Research Ethics Committees can audit ethical standards in research. *J Med Ethics* 1997;23:379–81.
36. Antes G, Chalmers I. Under-reporting of clinical trials is unethical. *Lancet* 2003;361:978–9.
37. De Angelis C, Drazen JM, Frizelle FA, Haug C, Hoey J, Horton R, *et al.* Clinical trial registration: a statement from the International Committee of Medical Journal Editors. *Lancet* 2004;364:911–12.

16

Informing patients about research

S Andrew Spencer and Angus Dawson

Introduction

This chapter is a short introduction to informed consent: what it is, why it is held to be so important in medical research, problems in obtaining it and how those problems might be overcome. Discussion of literature that might be useful to anyone involved in medical research is included together with advice about the composition of patient information sheets.

Consent and informed consent

Gaining the consent of patients for medical research projects has been an essential component of ethical research for at least 50 years.[1] As a result, it has long been standard practice to demonstrate compliance with this principle by ensuring that research participants are provided with a simplified summary of the research in the form of an information leaflet and that their signature is obtained on a consent form. However, rightly or wrongly, such an approach is no longer held to be sufficient and the focus is now upon obtaining an informed consent, rather than a mere consent, for a number of reasons.

Firstly, in the past it was possible to provide the information to participants and obtain consent without the need to ensure that the participants actually understood the details of the study. This meant that those patients who were not that interested in listening to explanations or reading information leaflets could still be enrolled as participants in trials. This is now held by many to be inappropriate. Supporters of such a view argue that all patients should be required to give an informed consent. Secondly, in recent times there have been some highly publicised complaints about the conduct of medical research. For example, parents have alleged that although they signed the relevant consent forms, they did not know what they were signing.[2] Again, the solution promulgated is informed consent. Thirdly, there has been a gradual move towards a consensus in favour of a need for informed consent via all of the regulatory bodies with an interest in research ethics.[3,4] Perhaps the most important change in the UK, responding to the relevant European Union directive, is the Department of Health's Research Governance Framework,[5] which was published in 2002. The common basis for these changes is the idea that research subjects are autonomous beings who should have control over their own lives. The autonomy of the patient is now seen to be the central issue in research ethics. All of these issues taken together have resulted in the requirement to obtain an informed consent prior to research participation.

If informed consent is supposed to be at the heart of ethical research, we need to be clear about what this term means. Informed consent can be defined as a decision made by a competent individual on the basis of sufficient relevant information and free of external pressure.[6] All of these aspects need to be met for informed consent to exist. In the research context, there are many reasons why this requirement may be difficult or impossible to attain and some of these reasons are discussed below. The central requirement is that patients are provided with sufficient information. The types of information now expected to be contained in information sheets include not just a full discussion of the possible benefits and any potential risks of harm or discomfort resulting from the research (including the magnitude and likelihood of any such harm) but also the aims, methodology, sources of funding and possible conflicts of interest.[3,4] The requirement to gain an informed consent is not only required by research ethics committees and the relevant regulatory framework but is also increasingly required by journals before publication.[7]

The process of gaining informed consent

Informed consent can, of course, only be forthcoming from those potential research participants with sufficient competence or capacity.[8] However, it is important that research is carried out in groups with no such competence, such as children or incompetent adults. Such research is the only way to improve the quality of people's lives through medical interventions. Where individuals cannot provide an informed consent, alternative regulations come into play, because it is thought such individuals are particularly vulnerable to research.[8,9] These guidelines should be studied by anyone conducting research with these groups to ensure that their proposed research project meets the relevant criteria. This will save time at the research ethics review stage. For example, in the case of an 'incompetent' child, it is important to make sure that informed consent is obtained from someone with parental responsibility (the father may not have this if the parents are not married). Where a child is competent and able to understand the process, they may be able to give an informed consent even if they are officially still considered to be legally a child. However, in such circumstances, parental support for the child's decision would also be expected.[10]

In addition to imparting the correct information, it is also important to ensure that the prospective participants are given adequate time to consider whether they wish to take part (normally 24 hours) and that they appreciate that entry into the study is voluntary.

It is vital that the process of gaining an informed consent is not just correct but can be seen to be so from the relevant documentation that surrounds a study. For example, it is essential to record in the patient notes the procedure that has been followed in gaining consent. Details to be recorded should include the individuals with whom the trial has been discussed, the length of time given for consideration and the date and version number of the information sheet given. It is crucial that consent forms are completed fully and correctly and are witnessed. The person witnessing must print their name to ensure that they can be traced should any dispute occur later. Multiple copies of the consent form are required, so that one can be filed in the patient's notes, one given to the patient and one stored safely by the investigator. Some organisations will also require a copy to go to the research governance office.

Anyone gaining informed consent should be trained in the correct procedure and chief investigators (the named individual responsible for the conduct of the study) must be reassured that if the taking of consent is delegated, then those undertaking the task are able to do this correctly. To this end, advice on gaining an informed consent has been developed which a junior researcher can be asked to sign to demonstrate that they have been made aware of the correct procedure.[11] Training courses may be available within trusts to help to develop these skills, as well as to increase knowledge in general about research ethics and research governance issues.

Problems in obtaining consent

Despite all of the above procedures, there is still a concern that it may not be easy to obtain informed consent even from all competent patients. This is because there is evidence that patients find it difficult to comprehend and recall elements of the research process.[12-14] For example, there is evidence that they often struggle to understand the reasons for randomisation and they can fail to grasp that proposed treatments are not always better than existing treatments.[15,16] Media reporting of miracle cures fuels this particular misconception. Patients' recall of the simplest event (such as being given an information leaflet) is surprisingly low.[13] It is important to note that problems with comprehension were found to exist in competent patients, many of whom were held to be able to give an adequate informed consent before participation in research. In the current climate, there is a real danger that such patients may be excluded from participating in trials, in the belief that they are unable to give informed consent. This may seriously undermine recruitment into clinical trials, with potentially serious consequences for future research benefits.

Another potential problem for the idea of seeking informed consent is the fact that there is not always adequate time to do so. Many of the regulations governing medical research have been developed by the pharmaceutical industry.[17] It may be easy to comply with such policy in a non-emergency situation such as a phase I drug trial, because participants will have ample time to think through all the implications. The situation is very different in clinical research in specialties involving emergency care. Neonatal intensive care is a good example of a situation where parents are often in a state of shock and mothers may be in considerable pain or sedated following an operative delivery. Research is often needed to investigate the emergency and early management of such sick babies. So how is it possible to obtain a fully informed consent? It has been suggested that research could commence with the parents having quite a limited grasp of the study, provided that further explanation follows and the baby can be withdrawn from the study at any time. Unfortunately, this commonsense approach to emergency situations has not been recognised in the Research Governance Framework,[5] so researchers adopting this approach could be open to criticism if a parent was subsequently unhappy about what had happened. On the other hand, some research ethics committees might be willing to support such an approach, particularly if the research was seen to be low risk and with high potential benefit to the participants. Sometimes other considerations should take priority over the issue of informed consent.

Can these problems be overcome?

It might be possible to overcome such problems if the patients or parents already have a good grasp of the purpose and basic methodology of clinical research. One attempt to achieve this has been the development and production of an attractive generic research information leaflet that can be given to all patients attending a hospital. This approach has been adopted at University Hospital North Staffordshire.[18] The leaflet provides patients with much of the necessary background information about research, well before they are approached about a specific study, using real-life examples of patients as research participants. The glossy leaflet, which features photographs of local research situations and facilities, is entitled 'Clinical research: why get involved'. Included in the content is a description of the process by which research studies are approved and the role of the research ethics committee. There is a section on informed consent and another on risks and benefits of taking part in research. Research involving children and issues relating to informed consent for children are also covered.

This leaflet has been evaluated in patients and in the general public.[18] It was found to be helpful by most participants. More importantly, most people reading the leaflet were able to answer questions correctly about various aspects of research and at the end many were positive about taking part in research. In devising such leaflets, it is important to keep the English simple, a task with which the Plain English Campaign[19] is able to assist. Once satisfied, they will award a charter mark. It is also possible to obtain a more detailed evaluation through the Centre for Health Information Quality.[20]

Clearly, the written word is not readily accessible to all and, however well presented the leaflet is, many patients will not bother to read the content. There are, therefore, good reasons for looking to alternative methods. One possibility is to use a video presentation, which could be played in waiting areas in hospitals and medical facilities in the community. DVD technology is now cheap enough to mean that copies can be supplied to anyone interested, perhaps through registration on the trust or health authority website. The advantage of video is that it allows real patients to tell their stories about research participation and this is more likely to gain and hold interest than a written statement of facts.[21]

Preparing the information sheet

Any research proposal will require the preparation of a comprehensive patient information sheet. This will need to be considered as part of the review of the project by the local research ethics committee or multicentre research ethics committee (see Chapter 15). To ensure that every relevant area is covered, it is advisable to use the format recommended by the Central Office for Research Ethics Committees and available on their website: www.corec.org.uk. This mainly uses a question and answer format to go through the study, with headings such as:

- What is the purpose of the study?
- Why have I been chosen?
- What do I have to do?

The recommended 'leaflet' has 20 headings and a recommended format for the consent form is provided at the end. The website also includes some standard paragraphs that can be used to help with explanations, so randomisation within a trial is explained as follows: 'Sometimes because we do not know which way of treating patients is best, we need to make comparisons. People will be put into groups and then compared. The groups are selected by a computer, which has no information about the individual: i.e. by chance. Patients in each group then have a different treatment and these are compared'.

The materials produced by Consumers for Ethics in Research (CERES) may also be useful.[22] Other, more comprehensive, publications may provide assistance in the preparation of written information for patients.[23,24] However, the researchers' obligations do not end once any materials are provided for the patients. As mentioned before, the onus is now on the research investigator to ensure that consent is really informed, and this means that the patient truly understands what is involved in the research. Of course, the degree of understanding required is unclear and degrees of understanding will vary between patients but it is not acceptable to allow patients to sign a consent form if they do not wish to engage in the process of receiving and deliberating about all relevant information about the study.

Conclusion

The current research guidance puts informed consent at the very heart of ethical research. Patient information leaflets must be developed with this in mind. It is vital that the correct procedure is followed in obtaining consent, and that this is adequately documented. Where research involves incompetent patients, appropriate guidelines must be followed. However, even some competent patients will find it difficult to comprehend the relevant information. One possible response to this problem is to seek to raise the profile of medical research in the general population. Informing potential patients/research recruits about clinical research through the use of general leaflets and video presentations may provide some benefits.

References

1. National Institutes of Health. *The Nuremberg Code .Trials of War Criminals before the Nuremberg Military Tribunals under Control Council Law No.10, Vol.* 2. Washington DC: US Government Printing Office; 1949. p. 181–2 [http://ohsr. od.nih.gov/guidelines/nuremberg.html].

2. NHS Executive West Midlands Regional Office. *Report of a review of the research framework in North Staffordshire Hospital NHS Trust* (Griffiths report). Leeds: NHS Executive; 2000 [www.dh.gov.uk/assetRoot/04/01/45/42/04014542.pdf].

3. World Medical Association. *Declaration of Helsinki. Ethical Principles for Medical Research Involving Human Subjects.* 52nd WMA General Assembly, October 2000, Edinburgh, Scotland [www.wma.net/e/policy/pdf/17c.pdf].

4. Council for International Organizations of Medical Sciences. *International Ethical Guidelines for Biomedical Research Involving Human Subjects.* Geneva: CIOMS; 2002 [www.cioms.ch/frame_guidelines_nov_2002.htm].

5. Department of Health. *Research Governance Framework for Health and Social Care.* London: Department of Health Publications; March 2001 [www.dh.gov.uk/ assetRoot/04/01/47/57/04014757.pdf].

6. Dawson A. Informed consent: Should we really insist upon it? *New Rev Bioeth* 2003;1:59–71.

7. Doyal L. Informed consent in medical research. Journals should not publish research to which patients have not given fully informed consent: with three exceptions. *BMJ* 1997;314:1107–11.

8. British Medical Association; Law Society. *Assessment of Mental Incapacity: Guidance for Doctors and Lawyers.* 2nd ed. London: BMJ Books; 2004.

9. McIntosh N, Bates P, Brykczynska G, Dunstan G, Goldman A, Harvey D, *et al.* Guidelines for the ethical conduct of medical research involving children. Royal College of Paediatrics and Child Health Ethics Advisory Committee. *Arch Dis Child* 2000;82:177–82.

10. British Medical Association. *Consent, Rights and Choices in Health Care for Children and Young People.* London: BMJ Books; 2001.

11. Spencer SA. Practical implications of research governance in paediatric research. *Curr Paediatr* 2002;12:232–7.

12. Kent G. Shared understandings for informed consent: the relevance of psychological research on the provision of information. *Soc Sci Med* 1996;43:1517–23.

13. Taylor EM, Parker S, Ramsay MP. Patients' receipt and understanding of written information about a resuscitation policy: report from New Zealand. *Bioethics* 1998;12:64–76.

14. Turner P, Williams C. Informed consent: patients listen and read, but what information do they retain? *N Z Med J* 2002;115:U218.

15. Snowdon C, Garcia J, Elbourne D. Making sense of randomization; responses of parents of critically ill babies to random allocation of treatment in a clinical trial. *Soc Sci Med* 1997;45:1337–55.

16. Featherstone K, Donovan JL. "Why don't they just tell me straight, why allocate it?" The struggle to make sense of participating in a randomised controlled trial. *Soc Sci Med* 2002;55:709–19.

17. European Agency for the Evaluation of Medicinal Products. *Guideline for good clinical practice.* ICH Topic E6. London: European Agency for the Evaluation of Medicinal Products; 2002 [www.emea.eu.int/pdfs/human/ich/013595en.pdf].

18. Spencer SA, Dawson A, Rigby C, Leighton N, Wakefield J. Informing patients about research: evaluation of an information leaflet. *Quality in Primary Care* 2004;12:37–46.

19. Plain English Campaign, PO Box 3, New Mills, High Peak, SK22 4QP.

20. Centre for Health Information Quality, The Help for Health Trust, Highcroft, Romsey Road, Winchester, Hampshire, SO22 5DH.

21. Dawson A, Spencer SA. Informing children and parents about research. *Archives Dis Child* 2005;90:233–5.

22. Consumers for Ethics in Research. *Health research and you: what you need to think about.* 2003 [www.ceres.org.uk].

23. Coulter A, Entwhistle V, Gilbert D. *Informing Patients: an Assessment of the Quality of Patient Information Materials.* London: Kings Fund Publishing; 1998.

24. Duman M. *Producing Patient Information: How to Research, Develop and Produce Effective Information Resources.* 2nd ed. London: Kings Fund Publishing; 2005.

17

Supervising and being supervised

David M Luesley

Background

Good researchers do not know all the right answers but endeavour to ask the right questions. The process of supervising research students should start with this philosophy, to encourage open thinking, critical analysis of data and to define the limits of their generalisations.

This chapter assumes that most, if not all, research supervisors themselves have experience of research. To be effective in research supervision, a supervisor must have both research and supervision skills. Given the above, this chapter purposely omits the other common problems surrounding research such as design, strategy, techniques and methods, reliability and validity. The objectives are those of supervising and being supervised and for the purposes of this chapter relates primarily to higher degrees (PhD, MD and MPhil), although many of the principles equally apply to other research situations, such as undergraduate projects.

Obviously, the needs of each situation differ and an appreciation of this simple fact is essential for all those who wish to supervise research. It follows that the relationship between supervisor and student is not prescribed. All 'research relationships' differ and the differences reflect the project, timescales, levels of academic excellence and, of course, the individual personalities of the parties concerned and how they interact. Nevertheless, there may well be some institutional rules in place that impose a degree of structure on the way research is carried out. This usually relates to regular appraisal or supervision. This is becoming an increasingly important component of funded research, as it is patently a waste of precious resources if the research process founders because of negligent supervision. However, as we shall see later, imposing too rigid a structure may be wasteful in terms of time and may also stifle originality and the development of independent thinking.

Why do people supervise?

Most students expect to have some degree of supervision, but why do established academics wish to supervise others? Again, this subject largely lies outside the brief of this chapter, yet it is important to consider it in passing, as it may impinge significantly on the relationship between the supervisor and the student. Academics throughout the UK regard research as a part of their multidisciplinary brief and, indeed, are to a certain extent assessed on their research output. Supervisors might, therefore, improve their prestige and academic standing by having many research students involved in many, usually related, projects. This might not be to the benefit of individual students in such a programme, unless the supervisor also accords similar high priorities to quality research education and completion of projects. Naturally, this becomes more difficult to achieve as one's work group or team expands and the wise supervisor should always consider the educational implications of research supervision alongside the benefits of high research output for the department. Some universities now impose limits on the number of postgraduate research students for whom any one supervisor may assume responsibility. At present, this does not apply universally. At one extreme, a student may gain considerable and valuable experience through planned and thoughtful supervision from a high profile academic. At the other extreme, a student may be little more than another pair of hands required to fulfil the supervisors overall goal of running a programme.

How types of project impact on the supervisory process

Projects can generally be divided into exploratory and goal directed phases. In the most simple terms, exploratory means defining the questions. It is involved with approaching new problems or issues about which little is known. The research idea can be less well structured at the outset. In some situations, this phase may occupy most of the time period spent in research. Other types of research or phases within a predefined programme are testing hypotheses (derived from exploratory work), problem solving (again derived from previous phases) and finally orientating towards a goal. In most postgraduate medical degrees, research is largely goal-orientated. A problem will have been identified and proposals to address the issue drawn up. The goal is then defined as various steps required to reach that goal.

Most projects will have an initial exploratory component and then a longer goal-orientated component and the needs of each from the supervisor–student relationship differ. The first phase relates to creative thinking and encouraging the student to be confident in developing their own concepts and ideas while the structured phase aims to take the student through the process of planning, data gathering and analysis to test the ideas originally developed. Supervisors should have a firm grasp of the relative components of a project and, with a knowledge of the skills and capabilities of the students, will structure the frequency, content and intensity of the supervision process around the student and the project.

Things to do at the outset

Choosing the right candidate

In real life, students may have little or no influence on who will supervise their research, although they may be able to influence who will not supervise them. Supervisors are either appointed by the research institution or self-selected by virtue of having obtained the necessary resources to undertake a project or programme. Prospective students should aim to work with supervisors who have an established research record in the field of interest and also, although this is not always possible, select a supervisor who has an established record in research supervision.

Similarly, it is vital for research supervisors to select appropriate candidates for research. The selection process will, to a certain extent, be determined by the nature of the project; for instance, if the project requires a significant clinical interface such as counselling and recruiting patients, then a candidate must already have attained a certain level of expertise in this area. Some new skills will obviously need to be brought in and latent talent developed. There is no such thing as the ideal research student, as each individual may possess varying degrees of talent or accomplishment in most of the key areas. These might include:

- the ability to grasp new concepts quickly
- analytical reasoning
- motivation
- perseverance
- organisational skills
- independence
- capability for original thinking
- self-confidence
- previous experience
- ability to establish good working relationships
  (adapted from Engineering and Physical Sciences Research Council).[1]

Understandably, any one candidate is unlikely to possess all of these skills and, for these reasons and because of the difficulty in accurately assessing such attributes, a process of informal interviewing, perhaps on more than one occasion, is useful. This will also allow the potential supervisor to gain some insights into what the potential student wishes to achieve and why they have been motivated to choose you as their supervisor.

Choosing the right project

This may seem simple but, in practice, choosing the right project is both difficult and essential to get right at the outset. In most cases, the student will have selected a particular department because the work conducted within it is of interest to the student. The student should avoid the temptation of taking on a project just because it is there and has funding. One concept that is always raised with regard to higher degrees is that of originality. That most clinically orientated projects contain something new is accepted and indeed vital for attaining a higher degree. It is unlikely at the outset, however, that even the most gifted research student can develop flashes of insight and inspiration. It is the author's opinion that part of the research education process is to develop and nurture the intellectual talents of students, in order for them to be able to continue with their own original lines of research.

Prior to embarking on the project, both student and supervisor should go through the plan in some detail to work out rough time frames and what skills may need to be acquired before certain tasks can be taken on and goals achieved. Both should make an attempt to agree at the outset what is reasonable and achievable within the time frames. Both should also recognise that at this preliminary review, the structure of the project should be seen as flexible. The supervisor should make certain that the necessary resources are available for the student to begin, as delays at the outset sap the morale of both. For example, a simple immunohistochemical study, planned as a pilot to a part of the project may be a reasonable starting point. It introduces the student to new methodology that is both important to the project and a new skill. Results are usually achieved quickly and this is good for the student as it makes them feel well-integrated into the research team and they will have a sense of direction and momentum. If, however, the necessary laboratory space, technical supervision and materials are not available, then a lack of energy can develop which, if not dealt with promptly by the substitution of another equally appropriate task, can lead to feelings of isolation and despair. For most clinicians entering research, there is a major culture shock and supervisors should be well aware of this at the outset.

This initial review may take place over 2–3 days, some time periods more intense than others. It is useful to use this time as an induction period, introducing the new research student to colleagues with whom interaction will be to the student's long-term benefit. Effort put in by both at this stage sets the scene for the supervision process that follows and also instils in students the notion that, although not necessarily the same type of structured work environment from which they have come (say clinical medicine), research is equally if not more arduous, as time management and self-discipline are new skills.

At the end of this induction phase, it is useful to have some kind of flow diagram or project plan on paper. Microsoft Project™ is a useful package to construct these and it allows back reference in future supervision periods. It also allows the timing of formal supervision periods to be placed well in advance to allow both the student and supervisor to make adequate time available and any preparations necessary for these (see below). Tasks for the supervisor at this stage are:

- setting the ground rules:
  - any rules that apply across the institution

- any rules that apply in the department
- health and safety
- what the supervisor expects from the student
- what the student can expect from the supervisor, department and institution
- determining which skills the candidate has and which will need to be acquired
- deciding how and when they will be acquired
- determining whether the candidate has other skills that can be developed within the scope of the project
- deciding how certain skills will be assessed (plan manuscript writing, departmental presentations)
- inquiring into the student's short- and long-term objectives
- determining the student's interpersonal skills, so that research 'buddies' can be introduced (this is a useful protection against isolation later in the project when the experimental work is at its busiest)
- deciding how the student's project fits in with the rest of the departmental research portfolio.

Dependence to independence

Students should attain independence as the project progresses. One cannot expect students to arrive in any department and be the finished product. The role of the supervisor is to facilitate and effect the transition. The speed at which this occurs varies according to the student, the project and the supervisor. It should be made explicit at the outset that this is one of the key objectives of research training and it should be kept as an agenda item at each formal supervision session. Most clinical research students will have come from an environment where work has been closely supervised and the emphasis has been on clinical training and the acquisition of clinical skills. The weekly timetable is usually fairly structured. Research differs somewhat, as there is an inbuilt desire to allow students to use initiative and take certain risks in the building of a sound intellectual and analytical approach. If each step of the process is outlined in detail by the supervisor with a fixed time frame, the student will not gain independence and will remain in 'research assistant mode' throughout the training period. To develop independence, the student should be given leeway to develop ideas and test them. They will come to understand the testing process and will also realise for themselves which new skills need to be acquired.

Too much independence is, if anything, worse. Errors in thought and planning occur and eventually the project will grind to a halt. One cannot just give a new research student the protocol and suggest that they go off and recruit 200 patients for an intervention study that could be a part of the project. The problems of recruitment need to be discussed, any background reading fully understood and then suggestions made. Any suggestions that are positive and made by the student should be encouraged, while negative suggestions should be debated and discarded (using constructive criticism), only after the student appreciates why the suggested methodology is bound to fail. This is but one of many positive interactive methods used to teach the experimental and analytical process.

What students want

Students expect supervision

Although perhaps stating the obvious, this is one of the most frequent criticisms that students make regarding postgraduate research. There has to be a close adherence to regular and formal supervisory meetings. Reference to previous meetings is vital to ensure that the project is on target and that, if not, problems can be identified early and remedial action taken. For these reasons, the author recommends that both the student and the supervisor make notes at each meeting, if necessary referring back to the 'game plan' and making alterations to future plans as deemed necessary and appropriate within the confines of the project. In at least some medical schools, the DM is not (on paper) a supervised degree. Rather, great care is taken to mention only the appointment of an advisor. It is, therefore, important that ground rules for the institution where the work is being undertaken should be established from the start.

Students expect the supervisor to be prepared

Just as the supervisor might expect the student to have any planned work available in a timely fashion, students have the right to expect the supervisor to be prepared for formal supervision periods. This should be both by having read and constructively criticised any prepared work, and in planning the next steps, if necessary by having refreshed their knowledge of that particular area of work.

Supervisors should be available to their research students

Formal supervision sessions apart, problems can and do arise in the intervening period and if the student cannot have access to the supervisor to discuss these problems then inertia might set in until the time of the next supervision. This is precious time lost but, more importantly, morale can suffer. It can be very difficult for busy academics to allow this degree of access, as they are usually involved in many other aspects of academic life. Indeed, the busy and established academic with an international reputation may be the focus for research students, initially for the right reasons but, when it comes down to ease of access, the problems become apparent. A way round this problem is by making one day a week 'open day'. The supervisor knows that this is the time when any of their research students may informally meet and discuss their various projects, while at the same time the students know that this is the time to make those informal approaches. One must stress, however, that all supervisors and students are individuals who may work in different ways. A mutually agreed method of access should be planned at the outset so that the supervisor and student feel comfortable and secure in the arrangement. One must try to avoid making the student feel that they are imposing on 'valuable' academic time, yet at the same time instil some form of discipline so that time is not overly wasted on trivia.

Students expect an open, friendly and supportive attitude

An open, friendly and supportive attitude is the basis of that underlying bond or relationship that research students have with their supervisors. Constructive criticism requires bipartite and open debate and not a one-way didactic process.

Students expect constructive criticism

This is often harder to achieve than first meets the eye. Everyone is sensitive to a degree and, in this situation, the supervisor must not intimidate, yet at the same time they should foster the learning process. Positive feedback and encouragement are required and not a focus on what the supervisor may feel are negative aspects. Encouraging reflective discussion such as 'If you were tackling that problem again, is there anything you would do differently?' followed by 'Why do you feel that would be better?' is beneficial.

Students expect their supervisors to have a good knowledge of the area of research

Often, towards the end of a project, the good student will have greater knowledge in one small area than the supervisor. During the process of arriving at this point, there will and should have been a period where the roles were opposite. At any point, however, the supervisor should always have sufficient knowledge to engage in debate and transference of ideas. This is another fundamental aspect of the research relationship.

Students expect their supervisors to have some responsibility for their futures

Nobody can guarantee employment in what is often a highly competitive field. Nevertheless, the supervisor should, at the very least, guide and support the student in their chosen direction. It is futile to make promises at the outset as a sort of incentive for hard work; the desire to work hard and achieve their goals must come from the students themselves.

Frequency and type of supervision

The supervision process can be divided into three phases:

- The introductory phase, when the supervisor introduces short-term objectives, work to be done and provides detailed feedback and constructive criticism.
- The intermediate phase is more support and guidance than direction. Goals are jointly discussed and planned and any work done by the student is criticised jointly.
- The final phase includes exchanging ideas, although the student makes the decisions regarding the work to be accomplished and the appropriate time frames. More detailed and critical analyses should be provided by the student without any prompting or suggestion.

The primary skill of the supervisor is knowing when the transition between these phases should occur. Formal supervision sessions should be scheduled, at least on a 2-monthly basis, but perhaps more frequently in different phases of the project, particularly at the outset.

Conclusions
Meaningful postgraduate research is both difficult, yet immensely rewarding for the student and the supervisor if the goals and objectives are clearly understood at the outset and if both are prepared to work as a team. Students should regard this as a first step in their intellectual evolution toward academic excellence. The experiences during this period, the highs and the lows (of which there will be many) will undoubtedly be a major influence on them and how, ultimately, they will become not only a credible researcher but also an effective supervisor.

Reference
1. Engineering and Physical Sciences Research Council. *Postgraduate Research: A Guide to Good Supervisory Practice, a Consultative Document.* Swindon: Engineering and Physical Sciences Research Council; 1995.

Further reading
Brown G, Atkins M. Effective research and project supervision. In: *Effective Teaching in Higher Education.* London: Routledge; 1988. p. 115–49.

Cryer P. *The Research Student's Guide to Success.* Buckingham: Open University Press; 1996.

Cryer P. *Handling Common Dilemmas in Supervision.* London: Society for Research into Higher Education and Times Higher Educational Supplement; 1997.

Delamont S, Atkinson P, Parry O. *Supervising the PhD. A Guide to Success.* London: Society for Research into Higher Education and Open University Press; 1997.

Phillips EM, Pugh DS. *How to Get a PhD. A Handbook for Students and Their Supervisors.* 2nd ed. Buckingham: Open University Press; 1994.

Okorocha E. *Supervising International Research Students.* London: Society for Research into Higher Education and Times Higher Educational Supplement; 1997.

18

Applying for a grant

Katrina M Wyatt and Paul W Dimmock

Introduction

The competition for research money is increasing every year with more researchers chasing ever-decreasing sources of funding. The determining factor in deciding whether a research project will be funded is the grant proposal. This chapter will cover:

- how to write a research funding proposal
- how to obtain ethical approval for your research
- the types of grants that are available
- the places to look for research funding.

Putting together a grant proposal

It is important to have thoroughly considered your project and have written a generic proposal before a source of funding is identified, as closing dates for research proposals are often only a few weeks after the initial call for grant applications. Remember too, it can take several weeks to receive ethical approval for a project and that some funding bodies require you to have received ethical approval before you submit your proposal.

The aim of a research proposal is to state the research question (quantitative) or area (qualitative) and to demonstrate how the study has been designed to address this issue. It will also need to clearly define who is expected to benefit from the proposed research. Above all, it must sound interesting and worthwhile if it is to succeed in the competition. Below is a list of headings that should be in every proposal:

- title of research
- summary/abstract (often in lay terms if the grant application might be sent to a charitable funding body)
- purpose/aim of investigation (the research question if quantitative)/area in which to gain a better understanding (if qualitative)
- background
- study design
- beneficiaries
- any consumer involvement in the project design or outcomes
- budget and justification of budget
- dissemination

- curriculum vitae of applicants (expertise of applicants and details of the project management team)
- ethics approval.

The background to your proposed research

This should contain a complete, up-to-date and relevant literature search to show the current state of research in the area. This could be presented as a systematic review of the available data. Give details of previous studies to highlight the need for your research. It is important to include in the background any pilot work or analysis that you have done which supports your proposal. Similarly, if a teaching package or questionnaire has been devised for the project, it could be discussed in the background and then included as an appendix to the proposal.

Study design

The study design is the most important part of any research proposal. This will prove to the referees that the applicants are capable of delivering on their proposed research project. The study design should include the following elements.

Setting

The setting of where the research will be carried out, such as in a hospital, GP practice or in the community, stating why this is a suitable place to obtain the patient cohort.

Inclusion and exclusion criteria/sampling strategy

Inclusion and exclusion criteria determine the people who will take part in the study and from where they will be recruited. Include a precise profile of these individuals, including their age, sex, nature of illness and so on (inclusion criteria). The proposal should also include details of who will not be eligible to take part (exclusion criteria). If the study requires control patients, the proposal should state who they are and where they will be recruited. A qualitative proposal should include details of the sampling strategy to be used, such as purposive or theoretical. It is also worth considering whether you will use negative case sampling.

Number of participants

A certain number of patients will be required to answer the research hypothesis. This number should be justified with a statistical power calculation. If the study is a qualitative one, you should state approximately how many people will need to take part, usually 12–15, and at what point no more participants will be recruited (data saturation).

Intervention
The procedure or intervention that is going to be applied to each person must be described. If the project is comparing more than one treatment, the method of allocation or randomisation of treatment must be outlined.

Outcome measures
The outcome measures should be clearly defined. There may be more than one outcome measure (primary and secondary) but the statistical power calculation should be based on the main (or primary) outcome of the study. If the study is qualitative, you should describe how the data will be analysed (for example grounded theory or content analysis). It would also be useful to discuss triangulation of the data and reflexivity of the researcher.

Data management
Describe how the data will be collected and by whom it will be analysed. Will a secondary analysis be carried out by a health economist or statistician?

Time plan
A time plan should be included in the study design with details of the milestones and when the project should have reached them. For example:
- 0–3 months, training in necessary methodology
- 3–20 months, recruitment and follow-up of patients
- 20–24 months, collating data, writing up project and disseminating the results.

This will clearly show to the referees that the timescale of the research and the project milestones have been considered.

Feasibility
It is important to demonstrate that the proposed research is feasible and that the numbers of patients or samples required for the project can be obtained within the given timescale. It will be appropriate to include any details of past success that your department has had in recruitment in similar studies.

The study design should also contain details of how the research can be generalised, such as what the widespread implications for your research are: for example, the number of people affected by a condition which the investigators are studying and how the research could impact on their lives and on the NHS, in terms of practice and health economics. If it is a qualitative piece of research, consider how transferable your findings will be to similar groups of people.

Beneficiaries of the project
Who will benefit from your proposed research? This should be the patients whose condition you are treating or monitoring but it could also be the NHS

if, for example, your research identified an alternative treatment which reduced the number of nights a patient had to spend in hospital.

Consumer involvement

If you have involved service-users or carers in formulating the proposal (they may have been on a steering group for the project or they may have helped with the research question or outcome measures), you should state this. Patient and public involvement is central to healthcare policy, practice and research. Some grant applications will insist that you detail how you have involved service-users and, if you have not, will want a detailed explanation of why not. A useful website for some guidance about involving service-users and carers is www.invo.org.uk/.

The grant budget and the justification of the budget

As the budget is almost certainly going to be cash limited, it will need to include what is essential to the project in order for it to be a success. Major items in a budget are often the salaries of the researchers, as well as any secretarial or technical support that the project may require. The salaries should include likely pay rises, national insurance and superannuation, which the finance department of the hospital or university should be able to provide. Other questions that may need to be addressed in the budget are:

- Does the research require a special piece of equipment or any laboratory consumables?
- Will the project necessitate any travel between hospitals or to patients' homes?
- Will the results of your project need statistical analysis or health economics analysis? A health economics analysis can be quite expensive but it could add credence to certain projects.

Other aspects of funding to consider are stationery, photocopying, postage, telephone calls and publication costs. It is important to specify the grade of staff required and the length of time they will be employed on the project. Specific quotes for equipment always add credence to a proposal compared with a rough estimate of approximately £X000 for items of equipment. The research proposal should also include a justification of the proposed budget. One of the things referees are asked to comment on is the financial feasibility and cost effectiveness of a research project.

Dissemination

The grant proposal will need to include details of how the results of your research are going to be disseminated. For example, conferences and peer-reviewed journals are two obvious means of telling the wider community the results of the study. It is now a requirement under research governance that the participants of your research are informed about the results and, again, they may have other ideas about reaching a wider client group, such as through consumer groups or specialist magazines.

It is important that the research proposal should demonstrate any collaborative or multidisciplinary approach to the research question; for example, if is there a statistician, health economist or social scientist on the project team. It should also demonstrate that the applicants have the local knowledge and expertise to carry out the research and that the study is feasible and cost effective.

Ethical approval

All research that involves NHS service-users and staff requires ethical approval (*see also* Chapter 15). An ethics committee is composed of lay people and health professionals who look at the research and decide whether it could possibly cause any harm (emotional as well as physical) to the participant or her baby. The ethics committee will only give approval for the research project when they are confident that:

- the risks to anyone taking part are negligible or minimal
- everyone agreeing to take part understands what is expected of them
- participants can refuse to take part or leave the study at any time.

Since 2004, all RECs have been working to a standard operating procedure. This means that there is a standard application form that is used by all NHS research ethics committees (RECs), irrespective of the research you may be planning or to which type of REC you may be applying. The form can be downloaded from the COREC website: www.corec.org.uk. The website also provides details of all the local RECs (LRECs). You will need to allow 60 days for a decision to be made.

The role of the LREC is to advise the NHS on the ethical acceptability of research projects which involve human subjects. The need for ethical approval now applies to NHS staff as well as patients and carers. Ethics committees ensure that local research is ethically sound and that the rights of patients and NHS staff in the study are maintained and that they are protected from harm. In order to gain ethical approval you will need to prove that the project is ethically sound and the research has potential benefit for the group under observation. The applicant will also need to prove that the proposed length of the project is reasonable and that any risk to the participants can be justified. It will also need to be demonstrated that the investigator is sufficiently qualified to carry out the procedures.

If you are going to obtain informed consent from the patient (and almost all studies will require it if patients are involved) then you will need to include a consent form and a patient information sheet with the approval form (*see also* Chapter 16). The patient information sheet is important, as ethical approval is often withheld because of problems occurring when the information sheet does not meet the required standards. It must be written in clear, simple terms and must tell the patient exactly what procedures they are going to undergo and what being part of the study entails. It will also need a state-ment saying that they can leave the study at any time and that their care will not be affected by this. For multicentre trials, ethical evaluation will be divided between multicentre RECs (MRECs) and LRECs. The LRECs have respon-sibility for decisions on local practical issues concerning the research. Overall ethical approval for a multicentre research project should be sought through one of the regional multicentre ethics committees, which, once obtained, will enable rapid local approval to be given.

Research governance is about the standards and defined responsibilities for the management of all research involving NHS patients, premises or staff. The Research Governance Framework was drawn up by the Department of Health in 2001 to ensure that all NHS organisations that are involved in research are aware of and take responsibility for all the research taking place in their organisation. It is now required that an approved organisation (sponsor) must accept responsibility for the quality of the research. It was originally envisaged that the role of sponsor would be taken by the funding organisation for the study. Most of these organisations, however, are not pre-pared to take responsibility for the total delivery of the research so, for most research, the sponsor will usually be the institution where you are based and will make a decision as to whether the research can take place within it. For some institutions, research governance approval is required before the pro-posal can be submitted to the ethics committee. An independent scientific review will be carried out on the proposal and once the reviewers are satisfied that the research is feasible, of good methodological design, answers a well-defined question or is of an area of interest, then the proposal can be submit-ted to the ethics committee. Depending on whether your proposal requires ethics approval before a decision about funding is made, you may need to seek research governance approval as well. Each organisation may have a slightly different research pathway for proposals and it is worth consulting your local research and development office about the procedures that they employ. Only when a proposal has ethics approval and an agreed sponsor who will take responsibility for the research, can the study go ahead.

Rejection of a grant proposal
Be prepared to resubmit your proposal to different funding bodies. If the grant is rejected, ask for feedback from the funding body to which it was sent; some will automatically provide written comments from the referees, others will give informal feedback over the phone. Also, ask for feedback on the proposal from colleagues who already hold a grant, if this has not been done at the outset.

Referees
Some grant-giving bodies ask you to name appropriate referees for the pro-posal, so it is worth spending some time thinking who may be appropriate. It is often unsuitable to suggest someone from your organisation (as they will be

deemed to have a vested interest in your being successful) but it should be someone who is familiar with your work (or the work of your department) and who is not likely to be applying for the same grant!

Types of grant that are available

Not all funding bodies provide all the types of grant shown in Box 18.1. Ultimately, the research proposal will determine which is the most appropriate type of grant for which to apply. However, for people who are beginning a research project, applying for either a fellowship or a project grant could be a suitable starting point.

A fellowship is primarily to fund your salary, thus enabling you to undertake your research project. Many fellowships are called training fellowships because they do not expect the researcher to have much, if any, research experience. A fellowship award will also fund some consumables and travel but, in general, it will not fund anyone else's salary. If the project requires additional technical or secretarial support, you probably ought to apply for a project grant. Although project grants are cash limited, they will fund all aspects of your project. It could be that the project determines which of the two is the most appropriate for the proposed research.

Funding bodies

Charities

The Association of Medical Research Charities represents 112 charities that fund medical research. It publishes a booklet which details the types of grant they offer and the amount they are prepared to fund.

Box 18.1 Types of research grant available	
Fellowship	A personal award made to an individual for their salary and some associated research costs
Project grant	A cash-limited award to enable a research question to be answered
Programme grant	Ambitious award to enable a series of related research questions to be answered
Travel and exchange	Funding to attend an appropriate conference or funding to permit a sabbatical in another research institution
Equipment and laboratories	
Conference/workshop	Funding for a conference or workshop to take place
Industrial collaboration	An award made to allow research to be carried out between industry and an academic establishment; funding is also usually required from the industrial partner

Research councils
The Research councils such as the Medical Research Council (MRC) and the Biotechnology and Biological Sciences Research Council offer all the types of grant mentioned in Box 18.1.

The NHS Executive
The NHS supports research at a national level. Applications are occasionally invited for support for research related to national priorities and these tend to appear in national newspapers such as *The Guardian*. Similarly, the Department of Health has a call for proposals in a particular area of health care. Research relating to looking at new ways of working, new roles for staff or new organisational structures are advertised through the NHS Service Delivery Organisation. Their website is www.sdo.lshtm.ac.uk.

The NHS Service Delivery and Organisation Programme is a national research programme that has been established to consolidate and develop the evidence base of the organisation, management and delivery of healthcare services. Another excellent website, funded by the Department of Health, is operated by RDInfo (www.rdinfo.org.uk) which collates health-related research funding opportunities from all providers both nationally and internationally in an easily searchable format.

Industry
Some pharmaceutical companies offer travel bursaries and small project grants. These tend to be advertised in medical journals such as the *BMJ* or *The Lancet.*

European Union
The key principle underlying the research the European Union funds is the fostering of cooperation between member states (the principle of subsidiarity means that the EU will not support research for an individual state). The research should, in some way, aim to improve the industrial competitiveness of the EU and must include at least three member states. The applicant will need to prove that the success of the project requires the involvement of several EU countries.

The National Lottery
The UK National Lottery does fund some medical research via the Community Fund but they only accept applications from charities and only one application per medical charity, so your chosen charity will only be allowed to put forward one proposal with your host institution (hospital or university).

Where to apply
When considering where to apply for funds, you will need to consider the level of funding and type of grant that the funding body is offering, as well as

the length of time that the grant will run. Another point to be aware of is how much intellectual freedom you will have; for example, if it is a drug trial funded by the drug company, ensure that you have the right to publish the results.

Lastly, some funding bodies, such as the MRC, offer a career pathway such that if you are awarded a clinical training fellowship, you would then be encouraged to apply for a clinical scientist fellowship and so on, up to a professorship.

Although competition is increasing and funds are dwindling, there is research money to be awarded. Probably the most important factor in determining whether your grant is successful is whether the referee finds your proposal relevant and interesting.

Box 18.2 Useful addresses and websites

Association of Medical Research Charities
61 Gray's Inn Road, London, WC1X 8TL. Tel: 0207 269 8820;
website: www.amrc.org.uk

Association of British Pharmaceutical Industry
12 Whitehall, London SW1A 2DY. Tel: +44 (0) 207 930 3477;
website: www.abpi.org.uk

Biotechnology and Biological Sciences Research Council
Polaris House, North Star Avenue, Swindon, SN2 1UH. Tel: +44 (0) 1793 413200;
website: www.bbsrc.ac.uk

Economic and Social Research Council
Polaris House, North Star Avenue, Swindon, SN2 1UJ. Tel: +44 (0) 1793 413000;
website: www.esrc.ac.uk

European Union Sixth Framework Programme
website: www.cordis.lu/fp6

Engineering and Physical Sciences Research Council (EPSRC)
Polaris House, North Star Avenue, Swindon, SN2 1ET. Tel: +44 (0) 1793 444100;
website: www.epsrc.ac.uk

Medical Research Council
20 Park Crescent, London, W1B 4AL. Tel: +44 (0) 207 636 5422; fax: +44 (0) 207 436
6179; website: www.mrc.ac.uk

NHS Health Technology Assessment Programme
website: www.hta.nhsweb.nhs.uk

UK National Lottery Community Fund
1 Plough Place, London, EC4 1DE. Tel: 0207 211 1800;
website: www.community-fund.org.uk

Wellcome Trust, Grants Section
Gibbs Building, 215 Euston Road, London, NW1 2BE. Tel: +44 (0) 207 611 8888;
Fax: +44 (0) 207 611 8545; website: www.wellcome.ac.uk

19

Communicating research: working with the media

David A Grimes

Introduction

Two centuries ago, Benjamin Waterhouse, a US physician, learned of William Jenner's discovery of the smallpox vaccination. Waterhouse immediately recognised the public health importance of communicating this breakthrough to the public. 'As the ordinary mode of communicating even medical discoveries in this country is by newspapers, I drew up the following account of the Cow Pox, which was printed in the *Columbian Centinal* (a semi-weekly newspaper published in Boston) March 12, 1799'. While the medium may have changed (to television), the message remains the same: the media are the public's principal source of medical information. How, then, can researchers capitalise on this fact?

Often unknowingly, researchers routinely address two audiences: the scientific community and the broader lay public. Few researchers today have the latter audience in mind as they conduct and report their work. Nevertheless, reporting of medical research in the print and broadcast media is a huge, and hugely important, enterprise. Research is of no use unless it is communicated. This chapter will describe the often tense relationship between researchers and the media and will offer some pragmatic (although unscientific) suggestions for developing a symbiotic relationship.

The importance of researchers for the media

The lay public and its media have a long-standing fascination with health. Its relevance to the individual is obvious. Interest in medical research is also keen. This stems not only from the hope for important breakthroughs, such as prevention of vertical transmission of AIDS, but also from a proprietary interest: in many developed countries taxpayers foot the bill for much biomedical research.[1] The public has a legitimate interest in learning the results of the research they have been collectively funding.

Highly visible medical journals provide a rich source of stories for journalists. In the UK, broadsheet newspapers such as *The Telegraph, The Guardian, The Independent, The Observer* and *The Times* all have at least one journalist who scans every issue of *The Lancet* and the *BMJ* for stories. They expect to find at least one story per week from these two sources.[2] In the US, health reporters for major metropolitan newspapers and the wire news services follow closely the press releases of the *Journal of the American Medical Association* and the *New England Journal of Medicine*. The latter casts a long shadow and is even the most widely cited journal in Dutch newspapers.[3] The competition for hot stories is keen and journals have had to set embargoes on news coverage to avoid rushed stories by journalists trying to beat the competition into print.

Journalists rely heavily on a handful of journals for two main reasons. Firstly, they believe (often incorrectly) that the most important research appears in these journals. Secondly, they trust (often inappropriately) that the peer-review process guarantees valid science.[3] The lead article in the 15 January 1981, issue of the *New England Journal of Medicine* was later retracted as fraudulent and is a famous example of peer-review fallibility.[4,5] Regrettably, negative reports that are unable to confirm 'breakthroughs' are not newsworthy. Corrections or retractions of flawed research generally get no attention in the media. Only scientific fraud seems to be newsworthy. Dissemination of poor science, whether due to misconduct or innocent error, has the same net effect: misleading the public.

The importance of the media for researchers

While researchers are clearly important to the media, the media are similarly important to the scientific community. As noted above, the media are an extension of healthcare providers in conveying health information. Numerous surveys in developed countries testify to this fact. Television is especially important. The average US citizen watches 7.4 hours of television a day. In the USA, the likelihood of reading a newspaper is related to income and the likelihood of watching television is inversely related.[6] The lower the socioeconomic class, the greater is the importance of broadcast media. Given this huge exposure of the public to broadcast and print media, researchers have an ethical obligation to communicate through them.[1] While television coverage is usually simplistic, newspaper and magazine coverage of health issues often presumes a rudimentary understanding of science. In contrast, large proportions of the public have little knowledge of science and its methods. The recurring reports of sightings of Bigfoot, Elvis Presley and extraterrestrials in tabloids provides indirect evidence of this scientific naïveté.

The media also play a key role in conveying medical information to researchers and clinicians. Like the general public, researchers read newspapers, watch television and listen to the radio. The internet is likely to play an increasingly important role as its use expands even further. It is not only the public who learn of research through the lay media; surveys of US physicians suggest that 60–89% sometimes learn of new scientific developments from newspapers.[7] One report quantified the impact of newspaper coverage of research published in the *New England Journal of Medicine*.[7] Articles covered in the *New York Times* received a disproportionate number of scientific citations when compared with 'control' articles that were published in the same journal but that did not have newspaper coverage. For example, in the first year after publicity in the *New York Times,* these research articles had 73% more citations by other authors in the *Science Citation Index* than did control articles without newspaper coverage. In contrast, when the *New York Times* shut down due to a strike, this effect disappeared. This natural experiment suggests that newspaper coverage itself, and not 'earmarking' of high-quality research, was responsible for the higher scientific visibility.

'Throwaway' periodicals (free publications supported by advertising) also contribute to the continuing education of clinicians. These have greater readership than do peer-reviewed journals, which are obtainable only by subscription or through organisation memberships. US periodicals such as *Ob/Gyn News* (a free newspaper) and *Contemporary Ob/Gyn* (a glossy magazine) enjoy wider readership than do *Obstetrics and Gynecology* or the *American Journal of Obstetrics and Gynecology.* Hence, researchers who want to communicate with rank-and-file obstetricians and gynaecologists may target these publications. For example, presenting research at certain professional meetings carries a high likelihood of coverage by *Ob/Gyn News*, which sends reporters to meetings. Similarly, after an article appears in a peer-review journal, some researchers write a lighter, derivative piece of about 1500 words for *Contemporary Ob/Gyn.* The magazine provides attractive graphics, an appealing layout and a loyal readership.

The media also serve an important role in research: recruiting participants. Researchers often use newspapers to advertise research protocols. These announcements reach a wider audience than do notices posted on bulletin boards in a medical centre. Drawing research participants from a broader population can improve the external validity (ability to generalise) of a study. A disadvantage of this approach is that readers of newspapers tend to be better educated than those who do not read newspapers. Hence, lower socioeconomic strata may be under-represented among participants recruited by this means.

Researchers' reluctance to work with the media

Despite the influence of the media, powerful disincentives deter many researchers from collaborating. Firstly, many scholars view colleagues who work with the press as self-aggrandising. Media attention may feed their need for visibility or simply be a ploy to attract patients to their clinical practices. Cooperating with the press, to some lofty academicians, is tantamount to getting in bed with the devil.

Secondly, a corollary of Murphy's law seems to govern interactions with the media: they have an uncanny knack of calling at inopportune times. Their urgent inquiries often correspond with urgent medical business already in progress. The reporter cannot wait; his or her editor needs the material now. They want to send over a film crew to tape a commentary when you are scheduled to be in the operating theatre.

Thirdly, many researchers fear the loss of control of their work in the rough-and-tumble world of lay media. Highly technical research is prone to misinterpretation by lay reporters and, unlike professional journals, lay publications do not offer researchers the reassurance of galley proofs. Some publications do, however, have an editorial assistant call back to 'fact check' and confirm quotations for attribution.

A fourth problem is bias. Publication bias is a major problem in professional literature: positive studies are more likely to get submitted and published than are negative studies. Thus, readers draw conclusions (often incorrect) from a skewed and incomplete database. Publication bias is even more acute in the lay media. Media tend to report positive studies and ignore the rest.[8,9] A *Wall Street Journal* reporter commented that this was not really a bias against negative studies but rather a bias in favour of positive studies.[10] A newspaper reporter admitted that 'selling a study that shows no results to an editor who doesn't understand science can sometimes be a tough task'.[11]

The net effect is the same: systematic distortion of the evidence. One example is the putative relationship between alcohol consumption and breast cancer.[12] Of 58 scientific publications during a specified interval, only 19% were mentioned by the press. Indeed, 77% of the lay press stories cited three scientific publications. No reporters referred to review articles on this topic. Stated alternatively, reporters ignored the bulk of scientific knowledge on this question. Another example with harmful public health impact has been print and broadcast coverage of the putative relationship between oral contraceptives and breast cancer.[13] In contrast, how many women have been made aware of the protection given by the oral contraceptive pill against ovarian cancer?

Bias can be even more overt. Reporters and editors may slant stories intentionally. An interesting variant of this is the balanced story with an inflammatory headline, written by someone else at the newspaper. Since many casual readers get no further than the day's headlines, the damage may be done with few words, such as 'Killer pill!'

Severe time limitations from reporting deadlines often produce unbalanced coverage. Reporters may have the interest but not the time to do background reading.[2] Their story may be due in 45 minutes. Research operates at a different pace. Few reporters will ask about or describe the rigour of research methods.[12] None the less, this context is necessary to avoid the overinterpretation of results.

Limitations in coverage (column space in print and time in broadcast media) can make adequate exposition impossible. Trying to condense complex research topics into a 60-second spot on the evening news is difficult.[6] Important information may be lost in the compression. 'Summarising a research paper in a few hundred words is hard enough, but having to summarise comments on it as well, with no extra word allowance, is even harder'.[2]

Finally, reporters assigned to cover medical research may not be knowledgeable in the subject area. Their editors may assign them stories on rotation. Thus, a common tendency is to look for the 'quick hit'. The measured pace of science is incompatible with this hit-and-run approach to communication.

Why bother?

Given these hurdles, why should responsible researchers get involved in communicating their work (and commenting on that of others) to the public? Consider the alternative. 'As long as the responsible leaders keep silent, the quacks and charlatans will fill the vacuum'.[1] Indeed, working with the press is an affirmative duty of responsible scientists: 'it is honourable to speak out to the press, to provide facts, to correct errors, and to give reasonable testimony on controversial issues ... If you do not meet your responsibilities, you will continue to subject yourselves to a selecting-out process'.[1] Having poorly qualified persons pontificating on medical research is painful to all reputable scientists. It is also largely preventable.

Getting started

Accept the rushed schedules of reporters
The inconvenience of disrupting your schedule at short notice will often pay big dividends. Thirty seconds of coverage on a network news broadcast may reach tens of millions of viewers. A 10-minute interview with a women's magazine reporter may reach more people than a physician could counsel in a hundred lifetimes of professional practice. The media become medical education extenders on a massive scale, in contrast to the usual one-to-one consultation.

Expect inaccuracies
Without question, the media will occasionally misquote or misinterpret a researcher, either due to an innocent error or to an intentional bias. This happens to all public figures and is part of the price one has to pay for working in this arena. Nevertheless, the benefits of conveying responsible, important health information to vast numbers of consumers far outweigh the risk of occasional glitches.

Volunteer to help
Newspapers, radio stations and television stations are often eager to find physicians and scientists willing to provide them with stories or to comment on others. To have a pool of knowledgeable commentators who can comment on research in women's health makes a reporter's job easier, especially given their tight schedules. Simply call the newsroom, identify yourself and express your

interest. This can provide excellent training in media for researchers and physicians.

For the novice, many medical institutions sponsor courses or seminars on how to work with the media. These media training exercises may involve not only internal staff but also journalists from the community. A comfortable way to make the initial plunge is with an escort: the media office of your institution. Many hospitals, medical schools and research organisations have press offices and public relations staff to guide researchers through the experience. These colleagues appreciate learning about new research of general interest, so that they can develop press releases and schedule interviews as appropriate. They understand well that favourable media attention generates philanthropy and more research support: success begets success. In addition, they often know the local press well and can anticipate likely questions and interview styles. They often sit in during interviews and can help facilitate the exchange.

Tips for working with the media

Few researchers have had formal media training. Hence, a few suggestions may make interviews more effective.[13]

Control the interview

Plan in advance what two or three points you want to convey. Regardless of what questions are posed, doggedly steer the discussion back to cover your key points. While this approach strikes the uninitiated as evasive, experience has shown the importance of sticking to a predetermined set of informational bullets. You can only transmit two or three messages in an interview; you should determine them, not the reporter.

Provide historical context

Medical practices or healthcare policy decisions should rarely be based on a single study, no matter how large or how well done. Reporters unfamiliar with the field often view a single study in isolation. New studies need to be viewed in the light of existing knowledge. When commenting on your own research (or that of others) provide the reporter with a 'discussion section' even if they only request a 'results section'. This involves discussing the strengths, weaknesses and potential biases in the research.

Explain the known risks and benefits

If a reporter inquires about the potential association between alcohol consumption and breast cancer, describe the protection moderate drinking affords against heart disease. Researchers need to provide the balance, since few reporters will have the requisite knowledge for balanced reporting. 'Faced with a strict word limit, journalists said that they found it impossible to include all the caveats and qualifying statements that are often found in research reports without killing their story.'[2] Unless researchers volunteer these caveats, oversimplification will occur by default.

Keep comments brief for broadcast media
Practice speaking in '20-second sound bites'. Because of the severe time limitations in broadcast media, lengthy responses are often unusable or are severely edited. Keep your comments crisp and concise; sentences of 20 words or less are easier for listeners and viewers than are longer expositions.

Use simple language
Medical jargon ('medspeak' or 'medicalese') may be lost on the lay public.[14] Use plain English equivalents, such as 'cancer of the inside lining of the uterus', not 'endometrial cancer'. Aim for English understandable by a child of 12–14 years of age.

Give examples
'If 100 women use the Yuzpe regimen for emergency contraception after unprotected intercourse, about two will find themselves pregnant at the end of the month. Without the treatment, about eight will get pregnant.' This is much easier to understand than saying that the Yuzpe regimen 'prevents about 75% of pregnancies that would have occurred without treatment'. While true, the lay public may infer (incorrectly) that 25% of women will find themselves pregnant at the end of the month, not 2%.

Conclusion
'Doctor' does not mean 'healer'. The word derives from the Latin verb *docere*, to teach. Yet 'doctor' is not a misnomer: only through teaching and communicating do we become effective healers. Physicians traditionally focus on the individual patient. However, our ethical and moral responsibility extends to the broader public. Communicating through print and broadcast media is a natural extension of our obligation to the individual. Working with the media can both improve public health and increase scientific literacy. If we fulfil this public responsibility, everyone benefits. If we default, the opposite is true as well. What gets communicated to the public should be not only newsworthy but also worthy news.

References
1. Altman LK. Communicating with the public: a physician's responsibility. *Bull Am Coll Physicians* 1976;17:6–8.
2. Entwistle V. Reporting research in medical journals and newspapers. *BMJ* 1995;310:920–3.
3. van Trigt AM, de Jong-van den Berg LT, Haaijer-Ruskamp FM, Willems J, Tromp TFJ. Journalists and their sources of ideas and information on medicines. *Soc Sci Med* 1994;38:637–43.

4. Darsee JR, Heymsfield SB. Decreased myocardial taurine levels and hypertaurinuria in a kindred with mitral-valve prolapse and congestive cardiomyopathy. *New Engl J Med* 1981;304:129–35.

5. Darsee JR, Heymsfield SB. Decreased myocardial taurine levels and hypertaurinuria in a kindred with mitral-valve prolapse and congestive cardiomyopathy *N Engl J Med* 1981;304:129–35. Retraction: Heymsfield SB, Glenn JF. *N Engl J Med* 1983;308:1400.

6. Dan BB. Communicating public-health information through the mass media. In: Council of Biology Editors Editorial Policy Committee. *Ethics and Policy in Scientific Publication.* Bethesda, MD: Council of Biology Editors; 1990. p. 247–9.

7. Phillips DP, Kanter EJ, Bednarczyk B, Tastad PL. Importance of the lay press in the transmission of medical knowledge to the scientific community *N Engl J Med* 1991;325:1180–3.

8. Proudfoot AD, Proudfoot J. Medical reporting in the lay press. *Med J Aust* 1981;1:8–9.

9. Koren G, Klein N. Bias against negative studies in newspaper reports of medical research. *JAMA* 1991;266:1824–6.

10. Bishop JE. Reporting negative studies in the mass media. *JAMA* 1992;267:930.

11. Neus, E. Reporting negative studies in the mass media. *JAMA* 1992;267:930.

12. Houn F, Bober MA, Huerta EE, Hursting SD, Lemon S, Weed DL. The association between alcohol and breast cancer: popular press coverage of research. *Am J Public Health* 1995;85:1082–6.

13. Grimes DA. Breast cancer, the pill and the press. In: Mann RD, editor. *Oral Contraceptives and Breast Cancer.* Carnforth: Parthenon; 1990. p. 309–22.

14. Friedman EA, Pennisi JA. Eschew obfuscation. *Obstet Gynecol* 1996;87:795–6.

20

Presenting a paper

Andrew Hextall and Linda Cardozo

Introduction
Attending a scientific meeting brings with it many benefits and, for some, represents a highlight of the academic year. Highlights include educational aspects such as learning new information, developing ideas, establishing research links with other centres, networking and keeping abreast of the politics of the specialty. There may be social aspects, the chance to visit a new city or even a new country, enjoy the local hospitality, meet up with old friends and sometimes make new ones. It is also considered prestigious to have a paper accepted, especially if it is for a podium presentation at a major conference. However, for the trip to be particularly successful, it is important that the presentation goes well. The following chapter gives some guidelines that will help make this outcome more likely.

Preparation
Even though a project may have been under way for many months or even years, it is often difficult to avoid waiting until the last minute to prepare for an oral presentation. It is vital that adequate time is spent planning your approach and making numerous revisions if necessary. Before you begin, ask yourself the following questions:
- What is the main message of my presentation?
- How long do I have allocated for my talk?
- Who is likely to be in the audience?

The abstract submitted to the meeting will provide a useful starting point and it is important to stick closely to the methods, results and conclusions included in it. Further help is likely to come from the conference organisers, who will inform you about how long you are expected to speak and the amount of time allocated for questions. It is likely that you will know if the audience will be of obstetrics and gynaecology specialists with an interest in your subject, generalists with some background knowledge or a mixture of healthcare professionals, some of whom may be non-medical, for whom the concept about which you are talking is entirely new. Try to pitch your talk at the right level, so that there is something for everyone in a mixed audience, without losing the main points of focus.

Visual aids

Slides, videos and props should be considered complementary to your oral presentation and provide a structured framework for both you and your audience. Most people now use computer-generated presentations, with a number of software packages available, the best known of which is Microsoft PowerPoint® (see Chapter 3). Check which version of the software is being used in the auditorium. If this differs from your own, dramatic and unwelcome changes in the layout, font and colour of the presentation can occur, which may only become evident when the talk is loaded. It is now rare for presenters to use 35-mm glass slides, which lack the flexibility of computer-generated images and often look worse. It is sometimes, although rarely, acceptable to use typewritten transparencies, but never use those written by hand unless you actually want to draw on them at the time – in which case, a computer presentation would now be preferable. The facilities available will also be outlined by the conference organisers but if you are in doubt or have a special requirement, telephone the conference secretariat or chairman of the meeting as soon as possible to make sure you get your preparation right.

It is really important to mix the text slides with pictures, graphs and tables to maintain everyone's interest. There are several rules to follow when making slides, which will improve your presentation tremendously (Box 20.1).[1] The temptation is always to use too much text to ensure that you do not forget to say anything crucial. This results in too small a font size being used, with too many words for the audience to digest at the same time as listening to what you have to say. Always try to design your slides so that they can be easily seen and read by people at the back of the auditorium, who may be some distance away at a large meeting. Use a consistent format with the title on each slide so that someone walking into the hall during your presentation will immediately be able to follow what you are saying. Make each statement short and relevant so that they will help the audience with their understanding of your paper and also give you a visual clue for what to say next. Avoid using 'flying bullet points' as this can annoy some members of the audience and distract from the message you are trying to get across. The use of colour will enhance the presentation but try to select the ones that project well.

Box 20.1   Rules for making good text slides (adapted from Lee 1995 with permission from the BMJ)[1]

- Apply a simple consistent format and colour scheme
- Have the same heading on each slide
- Do not use more than five colours (except for histograms or graphs)
- Use a large type size
- Avoid wide gaps between the lines of text
- Use short punchy statements
- No more than eight words per line
- Do not use more than six bulleted points

Everyone has a personal preference but popular combinations are blue/white and green/yellow. Always avoid using red text or pale colours on a light background, as these are difficult to read.

Data presented in a graph or chart is much easier to understand and remember than that given in a table. Follow the same rules as for the preparation of a text slide. Try not to include too much information and make the bars big enough to be seen from a distance. Graphs are easy to prepare on the computer and will greatly enhance your presentation. It is usually simple to switch between the different formats of data presentation, such as a bar chart, pie chart and three-dimensional diagram. In general, two-dimensional bar charts are the simplest form for the audience to understand. Although three-dimensional charts may sometimes look nice they are often more difficult to comprehend and your message may be missed. There is no excuse for using a table with a mass of data for which you have to 'apologise for this rather busy slide'. If there is an important point that you wish to make it is always worth reformatting the information, putting the P values in a different colour to draw attention to the significant results.[2] A simple but essential aspect of data presentation is to make sure that your numbers all add up and correspond to those in your abstract. It is worthwhile remembering that there is usually someone who will be trying to catch you out.

The use of video to show ultrasound images or a surgical procedure frequently pleases the audience because it aids understanding and may give a research concept more clinical meaning. However, this will eat into the time available for your presentation, so it is always necessary to edit it down to the most important parts beforehand. Hospital medical photography departments are usually very helpful, if given plenty of notice, and it is always a good idea to be as friendly as possible towards them.

One disadvantage of the need to load the presentation on to the meeting computer is the danger that others will be able to copy it, potentially infringing one's intellectual property. Make sure that the organisers understand that you are not consenting to any reproduction by loading your presentation on to their computer.

Oral content

It is a mistake to spend too much time making the slides for a meeting and to forget about the oral content of the presentation (Box 20.2). The slides provide a backbone for your talk but it is the way you present and discuss your arguments that is likely to win over an audience. To do this successfully, almost everyone needs to practise. Initially, you may wish to do this alone, perhaps in the lecture theatre at your own hospital or even in the mirror at home. It is then useful to ask a colleague or your boss to listen, so that they can identify any weak or confusing areas that need further work. They will also be able to help predict some potential questions, perhaps in areas that you had previously not considered. Use a clock or watch, so that you know how long the presen-

Box 20.2 Essential steps in a good presentation

- Decide on your main message
- Follow the rules for making slides
- Mix text with pictures, tables and graphs
- Practise until you feel confident
- Maintain eye contact with the audience
- Talk clearly in a friendly, relaxed but enthusiastic manner
- Finish with a strong conclusion

tation is likely to take so that you can make the necessary adjustments. It is important not to overrun your allotted time as it looks unprofessional, reduces your discussion time and is not fair on the speaker who has to follow you. Good time keeping is particularly important if you are the last person to present before coffee or lunch.

Sometimes you will be lucky enough to talk abroad at a meeting and there may be simultaneous translation. Remember than some English phrases are much longer when translated into a foreign language: 'John's hat' is ' *Il cappello di Giovanni*' in Italian. Other countries may not have an equivalent word for some medical terms or procedures (such as laparoscopy) and this means that the translator will have to provide a short description of the technique. As a basic principle, you can say far less if your talk is also being reproduced to a foreign audience, particularly if this is not being done on a professional basis. Translating your slides into the local language and presenting the same information in English can sometimes be a useful approach. It is always worth remembering that jokes can misfire when presenting overseas and they are, therefore, probably best avoided in this situation.

The first time you speak at an important meeting, you may feel more comfortable if you learn your talk 'by heart' in order to try to avoid drying up on the day. This will give you much more confidence as the meeting approaches.

The meeting

It may seem obvious, but you must leave yourself plenty of time to travel to the meeting, especially if you are going to an unfamiliar city or using public transport. If you arrive the day before, do not be tempted or persuaded by colleagues not giving a talk to stay out too late or drink alcohol, as you are unlikely to be at your best the following day.

Bear in mind the local climate or temperatures when selecting your clothing. Make sure you look good in a smart outfit with your hair combed.

Before your session starts, it is important to visit the lecture hall to get your bearings and look at how the console works. Check how to change the slides and operate the lighting and pointer.[3] Make sure that your computer disk or USB memory stick has been loaded and runs properly so that there are no last-minute technical glitches when you reach the podium. If you are using your own laptop, confirm that that the audio technician will get everything set up for you at the right time, particularly if you are following another speaker. If you are using glass-mounted slides, make sure they are kept at room temperature or else they may be spoilt by distracting condensation marks. Double-check that your slides are loaded the right way up and in the correct order. If possible introduce yourself to the chairman.

The presentation

As the time for your talk approaches, it is likely that your pulse will quicken, your palms will become moist and your mouth become dry. If this is usually a problem for you, ensure that a glass of water is available. When you are called to the podium, walk confidently on to the stage – this is your chance to impress. Attach the microphone to the lapel of your jacket and not your tie, as its movement often produces unnecessary background noise. Stand calmly, balanced on both feet with your head up and your shoulders back. Use the title slide, not only to introduce the talk but also to give yourself time to settle. Say 'good morning' to your chairman and the audience, introduce yourself and the co-investigators or participants in your study. Perhaps follow this with a picture of your hospital or institution. Try to have a friendly, relaxed manner, as this will often help to get a favourable response. This is also necessary when things are not going as well as you would have hoped, for example, when people walk in late or the pointer does not work. Always try to avoid appearing arrogant or over-confident, no matter how convinced you are that you are giving the perfect presentation, as this will alienate you from the audience who you should try to consider as your friends.

Your body language may be the cause of unnecessary distractions. To stop swaying or inappropriate arm movements, place one hand on the lectern. Do not flash the pointer around the hall. Eye contact is essential and you must look at the whole audience. Never turn sideways and start reading from the slides. Talk slowly and clearly, projecting your voice with plenty of energy, to maintain the interest of the audience. If you look or sound bored, the audience may react in the same way. Vary the tone, pitch and volume of your presentation, perhaps with an occasional pause to emphasise a point. Sometimes it is worth asking a question, even if you answer it yourself. Try to avoid 'err err' and 'you know' – be fluent in what you have to say. Be aware of your dialect or accent and make sure that you are understood.

Have something to add to each line of your text slides to ensure you do not just read them out.[4] Even if you know exactly what you are going to say with each slide, be prepared to add in comments which relate parts of your research to subjects which have already been discussed in the session or at the meeting. It is unnecessary to take a script or notes on to the podium. However, if you think you might forget essential figures that you cannot fit on to the slides, take a card as a memory aid. This is useful if there is a possibility that you will be asked technical or statistical questions in the discussion. As a general rule, you should use approximately one text slide for each minute but you may use additional picture slides or illustrations.[5] If your audience is unfamiliar with the topic or research methodology, use some link slides to make the lecture more easily understood. Carefully talk people through the results, even if they are shown graphically. Explain the axes to the charts, the scales, what each bar shows and then finally the outcome of your study.

Try to maintain momentum throughout the talk and have a strong finish that summarises the main points. The conclusions are important because they contain the 'take-home message', which is often the main thing people will remember. When you have finished, let the audience know by thanking them for their attention. Do not worry if you see a mass of hands raised to ask questions. This usually means you have generated some interest and is much better than having a silence, which may indicate that the audience was either bored or did not understand your presentation. Box 20.3 lists some of the points to be avoided in a presentation.

Answering the questions

If there are no questions, a good chairman will usually ask you something to get the ball rolling. Sometimes, someone in the audience will have found a particular aspect of your talk interesting and wish to have further information. Try to keep the audience on your side at this stage, even if you find the questioning aggressive or unfair. Thank the questioner for his comments, if appropriate, and then set about answering the question as you see fit. You will probably have anticipated some of the points during your preparation. If not, you should try to answer concisely while thinking on your feet. Do not make long, rambling statements that you have not thought through clearly. Again, try to concentrate on the subject of your presentation and area of knowledge. It is usually unnecessary to make supplementary slides that can be used to answer anticipated questions but it may be worthwhile if you feel there is a point worthy of expanding in the subsequent discussion.

Box 20.3   Points to be avoided in a presentation

Do not:

- Present too many ideas in too short a time
- Use overheads or a new technique at an important meeting
- Turn away from the audience and simply read your slides
- Make distracting or inappropriate movements
- Be over-confident, pompous or arrogant
- Use too many slides too rapidly
- Answer questions in a dismissive or confrontational manner
- Run over your allotted time

If you are unsure of the answer to a question, say so and perhaps highlight areas where further work needs to be done. Sometimes the questioning is particularly tough and you may feel that your supervisor should be involved. Although this may seem an easy option, it often results in the debate going on around you with thoughts of your presentation sidelined. Try to answer the questions as best you can without bluffing and only ask for help as a last resort. The chairman will usually recognise that you are having some difficulties in a particular area and move the discussion on. It is vital that your presentation ends on a high note and a debate taking place in which you no longer have a part is a bad way to finish.

Conclusions

Presenting a paper at a meeting should be an exciting and stimulating experience, often at the end of months of scientific endeavour. Although you will quickly develop your own style of presentation, it is important to follow some basic rules so that your talk is a success. Start to prepare well in advance of the deadline. Define the main messages you wish to convey, make the appropriate slides and practise until you feel comfortable. On the day of the meeting, talk slowly and clearly in a confident but relaxed manner. Do not be over-ambitious and never be pompous or arrogant. Use the slides to provide yourself with some visual reminders and the audience a framework for your study. Answer the questions succinctly, keeping a clear head and avoid confrontation where possible. Finally, try to look as though you are enjoying yourself no matter how terrified you feel inside!

References

1. Lee N. Illustrating and presenting your data. ABC of Medical Computing. *BMJ* 1995;311:319–22.
2. Thompson WM, Mitchell RL, Halvorsen RA Jr, Foster WL Jr, Roberts L. Scientific Presentations. What to do and what not to do. *Invest Radiol* 1987;22:224–45.
3. Day RA. How to present a paper orally. In: Day RA, editor. *How to Write and Publish a Scientific Paper*. Cambridge: Cambridge University Press; 1995. p. 144–7.
4. Mathers B. Ensure your slides put viewers in the picture. *Hospital Doctor* 2004; 4 March. p. 30.
5. Lashford LS. Presenting a scientific paper, including the pitfalls. *Arch Dis Child* 1995;73:168–9.

21

How to set about writing your first paper

Philip N Baker

Why bother?

Before starting your article, you need to identify what is motivating you to write your paper. You may have finished a study and feel that the findings are so important that they must be disseminated to as wide an audience as possible. Alternatively, you may feel that writing a paper will enhance both your CV and your future career prospects. Perhaps you need to silence your boss who is constantly nagging you to 'write up' a clinical finding. There are even some rare individuals who write papers because they enjoy writing. For many of you, there will be a combination of various factors motivating you to write this first paper – just reflect before you do so; does the paper merit your effort and will you be proud of the finished article?

Choice of journal

Before you start writing, it is a good idea to decide on the journal to which you are going to send your manuscript. The different journals require manuscripts written in particular styles and the choice of journal will govern the focus of the article. If the example of a study of a novel imaging technique in pregnancy were considered: a scientific journal would be most likely to accept a paper concerning the novelty of the technique, an article focused on the application of the technique to pregnancy should be sent to an obstetric clinical journal and a paper detailing the wider clinical applications might get into a general clinical journal. Unless you have a specific publication in mind, you should spend a few minutes browsing through the copies of journals kept at your local medical library.

The factors motivating you to write your paper will contribute to your choice of journal. In general, it is easier to get a paper published in a journal of low readership than in one which is widely read. Each journal has an 'impact factor' which indicates impact of papers published in the journal; that of *The Lancet* is higher than that of the *Archives of Gynaecology and Obstetrics*. You should be sensible: very few people have their first papers published in *Nature* or the *New England Journal of Medicine* but there is little to be lost by aiming high. If your paper is rejected, you can always resubmit to a lesser journal.

After you have made your choice, you should obtain the instructions for authors which pertain to that journal. Journals vary; some publish these instructions in every issue, others on a yearly or six-monthly basis. Most journals will also give these instructions on their websites.

Title

When you read some of the titles of published articles, you sometimes get the impression that the authors have selected as esoteric a title as possible, in the hope that this will dissuade anyone from reading the paper. Other titles impart minimal information about the studies they describe. You are not writing a detective novel; the best titles start the paper by detailing the major result or finding of the work performed. There are, however, ways of emphasising the fact that your work is an original contribution. In an article on how to write 'nifty' titles, Yankelowitz[1] suggested the following strategies:

- certain phrases imply soundness, such as 'A randomised trial of ...' and 'Multiple linear regression analysis of ...'
- some phrases suggest honesty, such as 'The failure of ... to influence ...' and 'The unreliability of ... in assessing ...'
- other phrases sound innovative, such as 'The pathophysiological relationship between ... and ... : a hypothesis'; and 'The ... factor: a critical new parameter in examining ...'
- further phrases indicate a timely study, such as 'The relationship of ... to urban health care'.

You should think primarily of a title that will aid your readers to find it when they search on PubMed or Google. Many journal publishers will offer assistance in composing a title and abstract. Sadly, some papers never make it beyond the title stage, so press on.

Authorship

Your next decision concerns the authorship of the paper. The question of authorship of papers can occasionally be a source of conflict and potential authorship is best addressed before any writing commences and, indeed, before the research begins. If you have performed most of the work of the study and are writing the paper, then you will generally be the first author. The senior investigator, who is supervising both you and your study, will usually be the final author. Other individuals who have contributed to the study design, the work detailed in the study and the writing of the manuscript may be entitled to be authors of your paper. The order of these authors should reflect their contribution to the study. Many papers list multiple authors and Quick[2] discussed the problems of having eight or more authors in his poem entitled 'Number 1 *et al.*':

It's 2 times 4,
And 4 times 2.
And what is more
Just who is who?
Assuming 1 is the driving force
And number 8 the chief, of course,
Then who is 5,
What did he do,
That makes him 5
Instead of 2?
Pity poor 7 and 6 and 3
Their place suggests obscurity,
In time's recall,
Said paper shall,
Be known to all,
As such and such by 1 *et al.*[2]

It is your job to ensure that all co-authors have made a valid contribution; many of the journals stipulate specific criteria for authorship. If you feel that an individual's efforts do not merit authorship, one alternative is to list their assistance in an acknowledgements section. For example, if a colleague simply allows access to patients, this would not merit authorship. It is also your responsibility to confirm that all co-authors have seen and approved a final version of the manuscript before it is submitted. Usually they will need to sign the letter accompanying submission or a copyright assignation.

Introduction

The introduction to the paper should explain why it was important that you performed the study. You should provide a brief background to the subject, focusing on the aspects under investigation. Although statements made in your introduction should be fully referenced, your readers should be able to comprehend your introduction without looking up the references. You should try to tailor the style of your introduction to the journal to which you are submitting. For example, if you are writing a paper on screening for Down syndrome, you will need to consider the importance of the details of prenatal diagnosis in greater depth if your paper is to be submitted to *Prenatal Diagnosis* than if you are planning to send it to the *BMJ*. Above all, your introduction should clearly state the question(s) you sought to answer and the hypothesis behind the study.

Methodology

The methodology section is often one of the easiest parts of the paper to write. It should contain a description of how you performed the study, with sufficient

---

Poem by kind permission of the *New England Journal of Medicine*

detail to enable any reader to repeat the study. If a particular aspect of the methodology has been described at length in a previous publication, it is appropriate to cite the previous manuscript and provide brief details. You should describe the measures that you have taken to validate the reliability of your techniques or assays. The exclusion and inclusion criteria of any patients studied should be described. Your methodology section may benefit from subheadings such as 'Specific methods', 'Patients studied' and 'Study design'. You may need to pay particular attention to the statistical methods described in the paper. If you have any qualms regarding the validity of the statistics used in the study, you should discuss these with your co-authors or a statistician affiliated to your department.

Results

The findings of your study should be included in your results section. These findings may be in the form of tables, graphs or written text and you should spend some time deciding which is the best way of presenting your data. It may be helpful to discuss the layout of your findings with either an experienced colleague or with somebody from your local audiovisual department. You should try not to duplicate the presentation of your data in more than one form. The results of any statistical tests used to analyse your data should be included. The results section is not the place for any speculation or interpretation of your findings; leave any such considerations for the discussion.

Discussion

Your discussion section should consider whether the study has answered the questions which it was designed to address and whether the hypothesis proposed in the introduction has been proven or not. You should consider the implications of your study; for example, whether changes in clinical practice are supported or whether further studies are indicated. This section gives you the opportunity to speculate, to extrapolate from your findings and to discuss your results in relation to the previous literature, highlighting areas of agreement and attempting to explain areas of disagreement. You may wish to identify caveats to the study, or modifications which, in retrospect, would improve any future studies.

References

The references section is an important part of your paper and you will need to spend time and effort to ensure that this section is free from errors and omissions. An author you have forgotten to quote or have misinterpreted may be the reviewer of your paper. Readers of your paper will rapidly become frustrated if they cannot find the references you have cited because of a typographical mistake. Different journals have different preferences regarding the style of reference citations and you should check that you comply with these before submitting your manuscript. The use of a reference manager software package will facilitate changing the style of your references should the paper be rejected and require a difference reference style (see Chapter 3).

Acknowledgements

This section allows you to acknowledge sponsors and collaborators who are not authors on the paper. It is particularly important for technicians with a major practical involvement in the paper or statisticians who have given time and effort to help you. Once the paper is published you should give them a copy of the paper with their acknowledgement detailed, as a useful way of retaining their cooperation in the future.

Abstract

Although the abstract precedes the introduction, you are probably best advised to defer writing it until the rest of the paper is written. The abstract is arguably the most important part of the paper as more people will read it than will read the body of the paper. Your abstract should thus be as clear and as informative as possible. The abstract also needs to be concise and many journals impose a word limit. Some journals require abstracts to be in the form of a single paragraph. Others request structured abstracts which include the hypothesis or rationale of the study, specific methods/study design/setting, results (including the results of statistical tests) and a conclusion (the 'take-home' message of your study). Your best plan is to read a few abstracts in a recent copy of the journal to which you are submitting your manuscript, to get a good idea of what is needed.

Covering letter

Once the final draft of your paper is finished and all authors are satisfied, you should submit your manuscript. This will usually be via a web-based submission system (such as that for *BJOG*: http://bjog.allentrack.net). Some journals ask you to include a letter to the editor detailing your submission and explaining why the journal should consider your manuscript; others request this information in a text box during the submission process. The letter should include the statement that the work has not been published elsewhere and is not currently under consideration by another journal. If part of the work has been published in a meeting abstract, some journals require that a copy of that abstract should be submitted with the manuscript. The author identified for correspondence does not need to be the first author; if you are about to move hospitals it will be more sensible to choose one of your co-authors to correspond with the editor.

Journals vary markedly in their response times. At least two reviewers will assess your paper and you can only wait for the editor's reply. However, web-based submission systems allow you to track the progress of your paper through the system, sometimes even into the production stages.

The response
Responses from journals can usually be divided into three categories:
- an acceptance without modification
- an invitation to respond to the editor's or the reviewers' criticisms
- a rejection.

An acceptance without modification
It is unusual to have your first paper accepted without any changes being deemed necessary by the editor or reviewer. However, if you do receive such a positive response to your paper, bask in your success but do not assume that getting your papers accepted will always be so straightforward.

An invitation to respond to the editor's or the reviewers' criticisms
An invitation to respond to comments usually means that your paper will be accepted if you can address the points identified by the editor/reviewers to the editor's satisfaction. Unless the letter from the editor states that a revision will not be considered, a detailed response is likely to be successful. You need to examine each of the editor's/referees' comments in turn. Some of the criticisms are likely to be valid and sensible points, others may not be so reasonable. In your reply to the editor you should detail whether you have accepted each of the referees' comments (making the appropriate revision to your manuscript), or why the suggested alterations are inappropriate or unnecessary. It never does any harm to compliment the reviewer when the suggested amendments enhance your paper. The editor may then accept your paper or suggest further changes.

A rejection
While it is disappointing to have your paper rejected, you should not feel too downhearted. Just as many of the best novels, football players and recording artists were initially unappreciated, many papers are accepted by journals of higher quality than the original journal chosen. Again, you need to consider each of the criticisms made by the editor and reviewers. You should revise your manuscript in the light of comments which you feel are helpful and constructive. After discussion with your co-authors, you need to choose a journal to which to resubmit your paper. The paper may have been rejected because it was too clinical or too scientific for the journal originally chosen. Your manuscript will probably need to be revised in order to comply with the journal's specifications. If your paper is repeatedly rejected, you do need to reflect whether publication is merited.

Proofs
Shortly before your accepted paper is published, the corresponding author will receive a proof from the publisher; this is often in the form of a PDF file sent either as an email attachment, or an invitation to download the file from

an FTP site. You will be expected to respond in 48–72 hours. You should read the proof copies and carefully amend any typographical errors. No major changes can be made to the paper at this stage. You do need to contact the publisher to approve your proofs, even when no alterations are necessary. Failure to approve proof copies has delayed the publication of papers by months.

References

1. Yankelowitz BY. Zany lessons for academics: how to write nifty titles for your papers. *Br Med J* 1980;280:96.
2. Quick DT. Number 1 et al. *New Engl J Med* 1969;281: 911.

22

How to write a thesis

Jennifer Byrom

Introduction

Aristotle said 'the roots of education are bitter but the fruit is sweet'. This is no more relevant than when applied to the writing of a thesis. Certainly, writing my thesis was one of the most daunting, not to mention time consuming, tasks I have had to face in my career so far. From day one of my research it seemed as though everyone I met was asking me: 'Have you started writing your thesis yet?' and for a very long time the answer was, 'No'. However, I did get it written and, once complete, it was not as bad as I had initially imagined. I, therefore, hope in this chapter to pass on some valuable tips on how to prepare your thesis. Unfortunately, no one can really tell you how to write, as we all have our own methods, but we can advise you on how to prepare and fine tune your thesis.

Before you even think about starting

The first thing to say about writing a thesis is that it is a big task – sorry, there is no gentle way to say this, it does take hours of work to write a thesis and so it should. At this point, I should also mention that there are no short cuts or magic formulas. Writing a thesis takes time, dedication, detailed preparation and if you want to get it done quickly, an iron will. However, do not give up yet, there are several steps that you can take to make the task easier for yourself, which will save time in the long run.

Dedication

Very few people finish writing their thesis by the end of their research post, probably because they are trying to get results until the bitter end, the work becomes all-consuming or they never get around to it. Many people take several months or years to write their thesis, especially if it is left until after they have completed their research and they are back in clinical practice. It is extremely difficult to write a thesis in an hour here and an hour there, as other commitments tend to interfere. It is easier if you write it without taking long breaks and dedicate time to the job. This may mean that you have to give up weekends, evenings or take a week off to do it. Think about it before you take on a research post – what a waste if you spend 2 years undertaking research and you never write up your thesis. Furthermore, it does not look good on your CV. No one can make you sit down and write it, you have to do it yourself.

Preparation

Before commencing any period of time in research, some preparation is essential. The first objective is to meet with your supervisors and discuss the project at length. You should be clear about the background of the project and what its aims are. Supervising and being supervised are covered in more detail in Chapter 17.

Once the work has begun, start thinking about the thesis. You may think you have months left before the project comes to an end but the sooner you get started the better. Careful preparation at an early stage means you will reap dividends later. Five things are required before you begin writing your thesis.

1. Become computer and internet literate.
2. Do a thorough literature review.
3. Consult the university guidelines.
4. Look at someone else's thesis (better, look at several).
5. Make a plan.

Computer literacy

I am sure, in this 'hi-tech' age, that I am preaching to the converted but the first thing you must do before you embark on any research, or indeed on any writing project, is to obtain a good computer with the appropriate software (you can, of course, choose to proceed without a computer but I am sure it will take 10 times as long). The next step is to learn how to use your computer. Either find a willing friend to teach you or attend a course. Many universities offer free courses to learn the basics and beyond. To my detriment, I was fairly computer illiterate and wasted many valuable hours simply because I did not realise that there were many useful aids available.

In my opinion, one of the most labour-saving programmes is an up-to-date reference manager, for example, Reference Manager® or Endnote®. For more information on available packages visit the Adept Science website at www.adeptscience.co.uk/products.

I used a reference manager and tended to enter a reference as I read it, which was easy as I was usually by my computer. You can also download a literature search from the internet to your reference manager, so you do not even have to type in the references and the reference, including the abstract, is stored for when you need it. The bank of references is not only invaluable for writing your thesis but also for writing papers, writing reviews or for teaching. Perhaps the most useful function of these reference packages is that it takes seconds to create your references for your final thesis. Believe me, I have written papers and managed a handful of references without one of these packages and it takes hours. You may well have in excess of a hundred references for your thesis, so it pays to handle them methodically and technically.

Other useful functions are those which are already included with most word processing packages. You can link documents and create indexes and lists of contents, figures and tables, again saving precious hours at the end of the process. Learning how to create annotated diagrams and figures is also invaluable. If, like mine, your research involves pictorial results, learning how to scan them into a computer and being able to use an imaging package can also be labour saving. See Chapter 3 for more information on computing.

It goes without saying that access to the internet can be labour saving. You can gain access to a wide range of online journals through most university websites. You may be able to view entire articles on many of the online journals and then print the articles. This is often quicker and cheaper than photocopying, can save hours of time rifling through journals in the library and can be done from the comfort of your own home or office. Furthermore, through the British Medical Association (or the RCOG), you can perform detailed literature searches on Medline or Ovid. PubMed is also an invaluable resource for literature searches. See Chapter 4 for more information on literature searches and on using the internet.

Literature reviewing

Ideally, before you start a research project, you should perform a detailed literature search about the background of the work. This helps in three ways. Firstly, it enables you to have an understanding of your chosen subject in more depth. Secondly, similar studies may already have been carried out and you may be able to avoid their mistakes. Finally, it is the first step towards writing your thesis. A thorough understanding of the literature relating to your research field is not only essential for writing your introduction but will also aid in writing your discussion. In addition to the internet, most postgraduate libraries will have packages similar to Medline, which allows you to search for relevant articles; their staff will also teach you how to use them. You can usually view an abstract on screen and then print it out. You can then search for relevant articles either in the library or via the internet. A word of warning about printing and photocopying – make sure you do it so that articles can be clearly read and copy all the references. I used to try to save paper by omitting to copy pages of references only to become frustrated when a key reference was mentioned in the article's text and it was missing from my copy.

Once you have started collecting articles you need to read them. This usually generates more references that need to be obtained. When reading articles, I used to have a pile of postcards next to me. On these postcards, I would write the reference and then any points/results that I thought would be relevant to my thesis. I would also keep references together in subject groups. This made writing easier, as I did not have to wade through piles and piles of references in no particular order when I wanted to include one in my thesis.

University guidelines and other theses

Most universities now publish detailed guidelines about how a thesis should be presented. This includes size of margins, page numbering and the use of abbreviations. It will also state how a thesis should be bound.

Reading someone else's thesis can act as a useful guide to structuring your thesis in terms of layout of text, tables and figures. The author is also likely to offer help and advice.

Your plan

I am a great believer in plans. I particularly like to have a list of things to tick off. If you make a detailed thesis plan, you can tick things off as they are completed and it can give you a much-needed lift. You should discuss your plan at an early stage with your supervisor(s).

Writing your thesis

Finally, you can start writing your thesis. You do not have to, nor should you, wait until the end of your research to start writing. The introduction and methods can be written as you are conducting your research. I wrote my methods first – this not only helped me to fully understand what I was doing but also helped me to get started, which is often the hardest part of any writing. Do not waste hours thinking about the writing process, writing anything is better than writing nothing. Once you begin to write, you often find that the words start to flow. The first draft is unlikely to be the last so do not worry about getting it perfect on the first draft. I then tackled the introduction. This becomes easier when you have completed a thorough literature search, read the articles, made notes on them and formulated a plan. Although you may not be able to complete the results and discussion sections until all the work is finished, you may be able to make a start. As each area of your research is complete, assimilate the results, analyse them and then write them up. This may already have been done if you have written a paper. Do not leave it all until the last minute. You may have forgotten what you did 2 years ago.

Results and statistical analysis

Whatever type of work is carried out, it is important that data are recorded diligently. I carried out a laboratory-based research project and kept all the details of my methods and results in a 'lab book'. As I worked through my project, I produced a detailed database, which not only included all my results but also my patients' details as well. This proved invaluable when I came to write up my results and when performing statistical analyses. A similar database is equally essential for clinical projects. This could be a paper database but, again, a computer makes the job less time consuming (make sure you also have a hard copy), particularly if you need to perform statistical analyses. Many statistical analyses, especially the more sophisticated, use computer programs to generate the results. While we are on the subject of statistics, I would advise you to seek the help of a statistician at an early stage of your research. They can advise you on what data to collect, how much to collect and, ultimately, how to present your data.

Fine tuning
Do not expect your first draft to be the final copy. Most theses are rewritten and shuffled around many times before being bound. Once you have completed a section, it should be spell-checked and printed off. Then read it carefully and check it again for spelling and grammatical errors before giving it to your supervisor to check and advise on how it could be improved. Before binding your thesis it is worth getting a third party, not involved with the work, to read it. They will often pick up errors that you or your supervisor has missed.

Referencing
As mentioned earlier, if you use a reference manger this can be a quick and easy job. However, do ensure that the referencing is correct. Again, refer to your university guidelines for their preferred referencing style. Reference your thesis as you write it and not at the end. It is easier to reference an article as you use it rather than go back and try to remember which article you referenced where. You should have a full copy of each reference used and should have read them all. I found it useful to keep my references in numerical order, particularly when preparing for my viva; my postcards were invaluable as they were essentially a shorthand review of each paper.

Putting it all together
You may breathe a sigh of relief once the writing is complete but you still need to produce the thesis itself. This is surprisingly time consuming. Check your university's guidelines for thesis production before printing. You should produce a list of contents and any figures and tables at the beginning of your thesis. Do not forget to acknowledge all those that have helped you, as the production of a thesis is rarely the work of one individual. Make sure your hypothesis is clearly stated and that you write a conclusion. Finally, after checking and rechecking you can print your thesis. Before getting it bound check all the pages are in the correct order and get your supervisor to do one final check.

Security
Ensure that all your work is backed up electronically and in hard copy. Keep up-to-date versions on a memory stick, CD-ROM or DVD – preferably in more than one format, just in case. Keep one copy in the laboratory or office and one at home. If you can secure a copy in a fireproof location, you could save yourself much grief. Theses have been completely destroyed in house fires on more than one occasion.

Summary

Writing a thesis is a huge and daunting task. It requires dedication and hard work. Seeking advice from others early is essential, as is careful preparation and attention to detail. Try to make an early start on writing your thesis and try to write as much as you can while you are doing the work. To make the process less painful, perform a thorough literature search first, keep detailed records of your results, buy a computer and learn how to use it.

Index

Note: page numbers in *italics* refer to figures and tables

academic careers   6–7, 229
academic detailing   78
academic foundation
    programmes   6
administrative interventions,
    guidelines   80
ADSL   23
adverse effects   74
adverse event audit   84–5
aetiological fraction   175
aetiology   167–8
age–period–cohort models   190
AGREE collaboration   77
agreement studies   181
allocation
    concealment in clinical trials   106,
        107
    random   107
amniocentesis   127
amniotic fluid   124
    karyotyping   131
    PCR-based diagnosis   126
analysis of covariance, gestational
    age   125–6
analysis of variance (ANOVA)   157
analytic epidemiology   162, 167–88
    accuracy   176–7
    aetiology   167–8
    association   167–72
    bias   175
    censoring   182–4
    confounding   172–4
    diagnosis   176
    discriminatory power   184–6
    effect modification   174

outcomes   187–8
prognosis   181–2
prognostic groups   184–6
validation   184–6
withdrawal   182–4
Animal Care and Use
    Committee   116
animal research   113–19
    alternative procedures   114, 116
    Certificate Holder   118
    ethical review process   116–17
    ethics   113
    facilities   115
    fetal studies   128–9
    Home Office inspection   118
    informing the public   118–19
    invertebrates   114
    location   115
    Personal Licence   117
    Project Licence   117
    reduction/refinement/
        replacement   116
    relevance   114
    species selection   114–15
    test data extrapolation to man   114
    time requirements   115
    vertebrates   114–15
Animals (Scientific Procedures) Act
    (1986)   115, 116, 117–18
Animals Procedures
    Committee   116
answerable questions   59–61
antibodies, validation   136
antibody assays   136–7
area under the curve   177, 185

articles
  derivative   232
  journal   80
aspirin, low-dose   128
association   167–72
audiovisual materials   80
  video presentations   209–10
audit   79, 83–94
  clinical   83–4
  criteria for good-quality care   87
  criterion-based   85–94
  definition   83
  fetal research   124–5
  multi-centre   94
  research difference   83, 196
  research protocols   203
  sample size calculation   88
  styles/types   84–6
author searching   49
autoimmune disease   132
autonomy of patients   206–7

Barker hypothesis   132
Bayesian analysis   127, 161
Bayesian trials   101
bias   63–4, 75
  analytic epidemiology   175
  data analysis   108
  publication   233
bibliographic databases   41, 43–56
bibliography   16
binary response variables   151
biomarkers   131
biomedical databases   *44*
Biotechnology and Biological
  Sciences Research Council   227
blinding, clinical trials   98, 107
blobograms   55, 56
Boolean operators   *50*
Boolean searching   34
Boyd Group   116
British Nursing Index   *44*
broadband   23
budget, grant applications   224

cancer
  clusters   189
  registries   165–6, 167
  statistical cure   186
capacity to consent   200–1, 207
capture–recapture methods   188–9
care
  criteria   87, 90, *91*
  patient perceptions   93–4
  quality   94
careers
  academic   6–7, 229
  clinical   6
  flexibility   6
  pathways   229
  structure   6–7
CART™   184
case reports   58, 75–6
case-base studies   169
case-cohort studies   169
case–control studies   58
  association   168–9, 170, *171*
  multiple logistic regression   174
  odds   153
  relative risk   169, *170*
  use   172
case-crossover studies   170–1
case-fatality rate   185
case-only studies   170–1, 172
case-time-control studies   172
categorical variables   150–1, 158
cause-and-effect diagram   181, *182*
CD writers   23
cDNA   138–9
cell cultures   114
Central Office for RECs
  (COREC)   197
Certificate of Completion of
  Training (CCT)   2, 3, 6
change
  confirmation of beneficial   89–90
  management principles   81
  measurable   94
  promotion   89

charities 227
charts, spreadsheet function 18
children
    influencing about animal
        studies 119
    informed consent 207
chi-square statistic 184
chi-square test 157
chorion villus sampling 127
CINAHL *44*
clinical careers 6
clinical effectiveness 83–4
clinical epidemiology 60–1
Clinical Evidence
    database 62, 69
    intervention categorisation *75, 76*
clinical governance 84
clinical interventions,
        categorisation *75*
clinical practice
    comparison with agreed
        criteria 91–4
    measurement of current 90–1
    repeat measurement 89–90
clinical practice guidelines 76–7
    implementation 77–80
clinical questions 30–1
clinical research training
    fellowships 5
clinical scientist fellowship 229
clinical training fellowship 229
Clinical Trial Authorisation
    (CTA) 128
clinical trials 96–110
    allocation concealment 106
    blinding 98, 107
    conflicts of interest 109
    continuing 40–1
    data
        analysis 108–9
        collection 108
    design *97,* 98–101
    economic evaluations 105
    ending 198

ethics 109
exclusions 107–8
explanatory *97,* 98, 104
follow-up 108
informed consent 109
interventions 102, *103*
outcomes 98, 102–4, 106
patient satisfactions 105
performing 101–9
phase I 96, *97*
phase II 97
phase III 97
phase IV 97
placebo 98
power calculations 105–6
pragmatic *97,* 98, 104
protocol amendments 198
public registry 203
quality of life 104–5
randomisation *97,* 106–7
results presentation 109
sample attrition 106
sample size calculations 105–6
statistical power 105–6
stopping rules 109
study population 102
subgroup analysis 106, 109
terminology 96–8
see also randomised controlled
    trials (RCTs); research ethics
    committees
ClinicalTrials.gov 41, *42*
cluster randomised trials 100, 168
clustering, space–time 189
Cochrane Collaboration
    evidence finding 72
    reviews of clinical
        therapeutics 70
    systematic reviews 73–4
Cochrane Library 51–6, 69
    combining searches 53–4
    datasets 51, *52*
    evidence finding 72
    limits 54

literature search   62
MeSH   51, 52–3
   results exporting/viewing   54
   search strategy saving   55
   systematic reviews   73–4
   textword searching   53
Cochrane Systematic Reviews   55–6
coding, data   145
cohort studies   58, 75–6
   association   168, *169*, 170, *171*
   historical   170
   matched   171
   mortality   169–70
   Poisson regression   174
   use   172
colliders   *173*, 174
commercialisation of research   202
communication
   informed consent   199–200
   media   230–6
compensation   200
computer modelling systems   114
computers
   budget   21
   buying   20–4
   fax-modems   23
   hardware   21
   monitors   22
   notebook   20
   operating systems   14, 15
   printers   22
   service agreements   21–2
   software   15, 21, 22
   statistical software   156
   thesis writing   253–4
   warranties   21–2
computing skills   14–15
   backup   23–4
   terminology   24–9
concensus process, local   79–80
confidence intervals   65, 154, 157
Confidential Enquiries   84–5, 125
conflicts of interest, clinical
   trials   109

confounding   64, 158, 160–1, 172–4
consent   206–7
   fetal research   122–3, 124
   see also informed consent
consent forms   225
   comprehension   194, 199–200
CONSORT recommendations   109
consultant posts   1–2
consumer-mediated
   interventions   80
Consumers for Ethics in Research
   (CERES)   210
continuous variables   150, 155
   association between   158, *159, 160*
   comparing means   156
control groups   75
Convention on Human Rights and
   Biomedicine of the Council of
   Europe   195–6
corporate fraud   202, 203
correlation   158, *159*
   intra-class   179–80, 181
   spatial   189–90
correlation coefficient   158, 179–80
corticosteroids, fetal lung
   maturing   128
cost–benefit equation, animal
   research   113–14
Cox regression models   184
criteria
   agreed   91–4
   good-quality care   90
   process   87
criterion-based audit   85–94
   change implementation   89
   confirmation of beneficial
      change   89–90
   current practice measurement   88
   practice comparison with agreed
      criteria   88–9
   repeat measurement of
      practice   89–90
   standards to be met   88
   topic   86–7

critical appraisal   58–67
critical incident audit   84–5
crossover trials   99
cure, statistical   185–6

data
  categorical variables   151
  changes   147–8
  discrepancies   147
  distribution   151, *152*
  double entry   146, 147
  interval   179
  missing   144–5, 145–6, 147
  mortality   164
  outliers   156
  presentation   240
  ratio scale   179
  registry   165–6
  reliability   150
  summarising   149
  types   150–1, *152*, 153
  unknown   145–6
  unpublished   202
  variables   150–1
data analysis
  clinical trials   108–9
  preparation   147–8
data collection
  cancer registries   166
  clinical trials   108
  format   146
  forms   142, 144
    annotation   147
  reminders   144, 145
  statistical analysis planning   150
data management   141–8
  analysis preparation   147–8
  backing up   148
  coding   145
  day-to-day   143–4
  electronic format   146
  paper format   146, 147
  preparation   142–8
  staff   146–7

  storage   148
data managers   147
Data Protection Act (1998)   142–3
databases   16–18
  biomedical   *44*
  design   18
  fetal research   124
  flat file   17
  output   17
  relational   17
deadlines   11
death registration   164
decision support systems   78–9
decision trees   184–5
decision-making,
    evidence-based   65
decisions, dichotomous   60
Declaration of Helsinki   194, 195
degrees, types   4–5
delegation   12
demographics of medicine   6
Department of Health   228
diagnosis, repeatability   179–81
diagnostic analysis   89
diagnostic tests   61
dialogue   61
discrete variables   150
discriminatory power   184–6
disease
  case-fatality rate   185
  cause   175
  clusters   189
  cure   185–6
  diagnosis   176
    repeatability   179–81
  fetal susceptibility   122
  late-onset   132
  prevalence   179
  probability   177–8
  registers   167
  tests   176
disease-susceptibility genes   130–1
dissertations   4
distribution-free statistics   155

DNA automated quantitation 131
DNA probes, validation 135–6
Doppler studies, fetal 125
double-blinding 107
Down syndrom 131
drug carrier systems 128
drug therapy
  fetal 128
  transplacental 121
  unlicensed 128
DVD writers 23

ecological level studies 168
economic analyses 59
economic evaluations, clinical
    trials 105
education, career research
    choice 3
educational materials,
    dissemination 80
educational meetings,
    interactive 79
educational outreach, guideline
    implementation 78
educational sessions, didactic 80
electronic publications 80
email 16
EMBASE *44, 71*
emergencies, informed
    consent 201, 208–9
endoscopy, fetal 127–8
endpoints, surrogate 104, 187
England and Wales National Cancer
    Registry 165–6
enzyme-linked immunosorbent
    assays (ELISA) 136–7
epidemiology 162–90
  aetiology 167–8
  branches 162–3
  capture–recapture 188–9
  clinical 163
  concepts 163–4
  descriptive 162, 164–7
  disease clusters 189

fetal research 124–5
  spatial correlation 189–90
  theoretical 162
  time series 190
  see also analytic epidemiology
equivalence trials 101
error, unit of analysis 109
ethical analysis of research 194–5
ethical approval 225–6
ethical review process
  animal studies 116–17
  external 193–4
ethics
  animal research 113
  clinical trials 109
  definition 193
  fetal 122–4
  guidelines 195–6
  informed consent 206
  intervention studies 172
  quality of science 115
  research 193–4
  situational 194
ethics committees *see* research ethics
    committees
EudraCT European database 203
European Union
  Directive 2001/20/EC 197
  funding 228
evidence 61
  application 74–6
  appraising 72–4
  finding 71–2
  grading/levels *74, 75,* 76
  levels *75,* 76
  literature searching 62
  media distortion 233
  relevance 74
  research 61–2
  strength 65, *74, 75*
evidence-based decisions 65
evidence-based learning,
    elements *70*
evidence-based medicine 69–81

definition   70, 71
essentials   71
evidence
   application   74–6
   appraisal   72–4
   finding   71–2
impact evaluation   76
question formulation   71
evidence-based practice   61, 66–7
experimental design, statistics   115

factorial trial design   99
fax-modems   23
feedback, guideline
   implementation   79
fellowship   227, 229
fetal blood sampling   126
fetal endoscopy   127–8
fetal gene therapy   130
fetal membranes   124
fetal research   121–32
   animal studies   128–9
   audit   124–5
   clinical   124–8
   consent   122–3, 124
   dead fetuses   123–4
   diagnostic procedures   127
   drug therapy   128
   epidemiology   124–5
   ethics   122–4
   field   121–2
   invasive procedures   126–8
   laboratory   128–32
   live fetuses   123
   molecular biology   130–2
   observational   125–6
   randomised controlled
      trials   127–8
fetal stem cells   129–30
fetal tissues   122–3
fetal wellbeing tests   126
fetomaternal cell trafficking   132
fetoscopic laser ablation   127–8
flexibility of careers   6

fluorescent *in situ* hybridization
   (FISH)   131
folate, periconceptual   128
format checkers   15
FRAME (Fund for the Replacement
   of Animals in Medical
   Research)   114
fraud   201–3
   detection   202–3
   peer-review fallibility   231
   prevention   202–3
funding
   applications   228
   bodies   227–9

gateways   35–41
gene therapy, fetal   130
General Medical Council
   (GMC)   196
Geneva Foundation for Medical
   Education and Research
   (GFMER)   38–9
gestational age   125–6
goal setting   9
good clinical practice, research
   governance   109
Google™   32–5
   Advanced search option   34, 35
   image search   34
   Scholar   33, 34
grant applications   221–9
   beneficiaries   223
   budget   224
   consumer involvement   224
   dissemination of research   224
   ethical approval   225–6
   referees   226–7
   rejection   226
   service-users   224
   study design   222–3
grant proposals   222–6
grants, types   227
guidelines   40, 59
   administrative interventions   80

clinical practice   76–7
  implementation   77–80
critical appraisal   77
development   76–7
ethics   195–6
implementation   77–80
incentives   80
penalties   80

hazard   183
hazard ratio   169, 184
health, self-reported   105
health statistics sources   166
hiding   13
HMIC database   *44*
Human Tissue Act (2004)   122–3,
  201
human tissues   201
hypothesis testing   154
hypothesis-generating exercises   109

imaging packages   254
immunoassays   136–7
immunohistochemistry   136
  antigen localisation   139
in utero transplantation of stem
  cells   130
incentives, guidelines   80
indomethacin   128
information
  for patients   208–10
  quality on websites   35
information leaflet for patients   209
informed consent   199–200, 206–11
  capacity   200–1, 207
  clinical trials   109
  competence   207
  consent forms   225
    comprehension   194, 199–200
  delegation   208
  emergencies   201, 208–9
  ethics   206
  problems   208–9
  process of gaining   207–8

records   207–8
  taking   208
  training   208
informing patients about
  research   206–11
intention to treat   108
interactive educational meetings   79
International Committee of Medical
  Journal Editors   203
internet   16
  access   23, 254
  literature searching   31–2, 253
  medical information   231
inter-twin transfusion   125
interval data   179
intervention studies, ethics   172
interventions
  categorisation   *75*
  clinical trials   102, *103*
intrauterine events in late-onset
  disease   132
Intute: Health and Life Sciences   36
ISP (internet service provider)   23

journalistic reviews   59
journals
  articles   80
  choice for paper writing   245–6
  impact factors   245
  online   254
  paper submission   249–50
  registration of trials   203
  sources for journalists   230–1
  title searching   49
just-in-time reminders   79

Kaplan–Meier estimator   183
kappa statistic   179–81
  weighted   181
Kell blood group typing   131
Kruskal–Wallis test   157

laboratory research   135–40
  fetal   128–32

validation
    of probes/antibodies   135–6
labour, consent during   201
legal capacity   200
life tables   165
likelihood ratio   178
linear predictor   173–4, 184
linear regression   158, *160*
liposomes   128
literature reviews   5, 254
literature searching   30–57, 62
    downloading from internet   253
    gateways   35–41
    general resources   31–5
    guidelines   40
    internet   31–2, 253
    medical search engines   35–41
    portals   35–41
    question formulation   30–1
    statistics   41, *43*
    thesis writing   253, 254
local concensus process   79–80
local opinion leaders   79
logistic regression   190
log-linear modelling   188

MALDI-TOF   131
Mann–Whitney test   157
Mantel–Haenszel method   158
mass media campaigns   79
mass spectrometry   131
matching   173
mean, statistical   155
    comparing   156–7
media
    campaigns   79
    communicating research   230–6
    coverage limitations   233–4
    example use   236
    explaining animal research   119
    importance for researchers   231–2
    inaccuracies   234
    language use   236
    medical information   231

misinterpretation of research   233
researcher
    importance   230–1
    reluctance   232–4
    rushed schedules   234
    time pressures   233
    training on working with   235
    volunteer recruitment   232
median, statistical   155
Medical Research Council
        (MRC)   227
    career pathways   229
Medical Subject Headings (MeSH)
    Cochrane Library   51, 52–3
    hierarchy   *47*
    Medline   45, 46, *47*
Medicines Licensing Act (1968)   128
Medline   33, 41, 43–51
    accessing   43–4
    author searching   49
    combined searches   49–50
    evidence finding   71
    explode   46–7
    focus   45–6
    journal title searching   49
    limits   50
    literature search   62, 254
    results manager/viewing   50
    search history saving   51
    subject searching   44–5
    textword searching   47–8
mental capacity   200–1, 207
mesenchymal stem cells   130
messenger RNA (mRNA),
        Northern blotting   137–8
meta-analyses   5, 59, 161
methods section, evaluation   63–5
microchimerism   132
Microsoft PowerPoint®   20, 239
Microsoft Windows®   14, 15
microvillus membrane
        preparations   129
middle cerebral artery, fetal peak
        systolic velocity   125

miscarriage 121
modernising medical careers 6
molecular biology, fetal 130–2
morbidity 165–6
mortality
  age-adjusted 165
  cohort studies 169–70
  crude rates 165
  data 164
  rates 164–5
mouse models 129
multifacted interventions 79
multiple logistic regression 173–4
multiple regression analysis 160–1
multivariate analysis 158, 160–1

National Centre for the 3Rs 116
National Guideline Clearinghouse
  (NGC) 40, *41*
National Institute for Clinical
  Excellence (NICE), evidence
  strength *74, 75, 76*
National Library for Health 37–8
National Lottery 228
National Research Register 41, *42*
newspapers 231–2
NHS Centre for Reviews and
  Dissemination 89
NHS Executive 228
NHS National Library for
  Health 37–8
NHS Service Delivery and
  Organisation Programme 228
non-parametric statistics 155, 157
normal distribution 151, *152*
Northern blotting 137–8
nucleic acid detection, fetal 131
null hypothesis 154
numbers needed to treat
  (NNTs) 65, *66*

obstetric cholestasis 130–1
odds 151, 153, 163, 164
  posterior 178

prior 178, 179
odds ratio 153, 157
  correction 172
  exposure *170*
  multiple logistic regression 174
Office for National Statistics
  (ONS) 164, 165–6
OMNI 36
  guidelines 40
opinion leaders, local 79
outcomes 182, 187–8
  clinical 103–4
  clinical trials 98, 102–4, 106
  ethical analysis of research 194–5
  measures 223
  surrogate endpoints 187
outliers 156
overhead projectors 19
Ovid *45, 46*
  literature search 254
  MeSH hierarchy *47*
  search history syntax *48*
  textword searching 48
  wildcards 48, *49*

paper presentation 238–44
  conclusions 243
  delivery 242–3
  oral content 240–1
  preparation 238–41
  questions 243–4
  scientific meeting 241–4
  translation 240
  visual aids 239–40
paper writing 245–51
  abstract 249
  acknowledgements 249
  authorship 246–7
  co-authorship 246–7
  covering letter 249
  discussion 248
  introduction 247
  journal choice 245–6
  methodology 247–8

proofs 250–1
references 248–9
rejection 251
results 248
submission 249
title 245–6
parallel group trials
multiple-arm 98–9
two-arm 98
parametric statistics 155
pathognomic tests 176
patient(s)
autonomy 206–7
information materials 208–10
informing about research 206–11
involvement 224
mental capacity 200–1, 207
satisfaction in clinical trials 105
patient preference trials 100–1
peer-review 231
penalties, guidelines 80
periodicals
throwaway 232
see also journals; newspapers
phamacogenomics 122
pharmaceutical companies 228
PICO-type questions 30–1
pilot studies 146
placebo, clinical trials 98
placental studies 124, 129–30
placental vascular anastomoses, laser
ablation 127–8
planning research 8–9
saving time 11
point estimate of effect size 65
Poisson regression 174, 190
Polkinghorne Committee
report 122, 123–4
polymerase chain reaction
(PCR) 138–9
amniotic fluid studies 126
real-time 131
population attributable risk 175
population estimates 164

portals 35–41
positive predictive value 178
posterior odds 178
power, statistical 64, 154–5
power calculations, clinical
trials 105–6
pre-eclampsia, prediction 125
pregnancy registers 167
prenatal diagnosis 122
karyotyping 131
presentation packages 19–20
press releases 231
preterm labour
investigations 126
prediction 125
prevalence 164
disease 179
printers 22
prior beliefs 101
prior distribution 101, 161
prior odds 178, 179
prioritisation 10
probability (P value) 154, 156, 157
disease 177–8
posterior 178
process criteria 87
procrastination 12
prognosis 62, 181–2
prognostic groups 184–6
prognostic index 184, 185
project grants 227
projection facilities 20
proportions, comparing 157–8
proteomic techniques 131
PsycINFO 44
public
information about animal
studies 118–19
involvement 224
public health 62
publication 3–4
bias 233
derivative articles 232
see also journals; paper writing

PubMed 33
  evidence finding 71
  literature search 254

quality adjusted life-year
  (QALY) 188
quality of life 187–8
  clinical trials 104–5
  self-reported 105
quasi-randomised trials 100
questionnaires
  missing data 144–5
  quality of life 104–5
questions
  answerable 59–61
  clinical 30–1
  data requirements 141–2
  formulation 71
  research *72*
  research evidence 61
  response rate 145
  three-part 60
  unfocused 31

radioimmunoassays (RIA) 136–7
randomisation
  block 106
  clinical trials 106–7
  explanation to
    participants 199–200
  stratified 106–7
randomised controlled trials
  (RCTs) 58, 69, 96–110
  association 168, *169*
  classification 96–8
  fetal research 127–8
  research design 73
  see also research ethics committees
rare effects 74
ratio scale data 179
RDInfor 228
receiver operating characteristic
  (ROC) plot 177, *178*
recruitment 232

referees, grant applications 226–7
reference manager program 16,
  253, 256
reflection 61
registers 167
  clinical trials 203
registry data 165–6
regression 158, *160*
relative risk 153, 157, 164, 167
  association measurement 172
  case–control study 169, *170*
  variables 184
reliability coefficient 180
reminder tools 78–9
research
  aims 3–5
  audit difference 83, 196
  background 222–3
  barriers to getting into
    practice 81
  design 72, 73
  dissemination 224
  duty-based 194, 195
  feasibility 223
  findings into practice 76–7, 81
  goal-based 194–5
  methods evaluation 63–5
  multi-site 198, 225
  pilot studies 146
  progress reports 198
  reasons for 1–3
  resources 216
  rights-based 194, 195
  skills 216, 217
  subject choice 5
  subspecialty training
    programmes 3
  time frames 216
  timing 6–7
  see also informed consent
research councils 228
Research Defence Society 119
research ethics committees 196–7
  approval of project 225–6

audit of research protocols   203
composition   197–8
emergency informed
      consent   209
local   197
operating procedures   197–9
progress reports   198, 203
protocol amendments   198
registration of proposals   203
submission process   198
research evidence   61–2
research governance   109, 226
Research Governance
      Framework   209
research literature
   critical appraisal   58–67
   primary   58–9
   secondary   59
research project
   choice   215–17
   plan   216–17
   types   214
research proposals,
      registration   203
researchers
   media relations   230–2
   recruitment   232
   reluctance to work with
         media   232–4
   volunteering with media   234–5
   working with media   234–6
response variable   151, 155
results, reliability   150
RhD typing   131
risk   151, 153, 163, 164
   cumulative   165
   excess   167
   unpublished data   202
Royal College of Obstetricians and
      Gynaecologists
   guidelines on disposal of fetal
         tissue   123
   website statistics   *43*
Royal Colleges, Membership   1

sample size calculation
   audit   88
   clinical trials   105–6
science
   poor   231
   quality   115
Science Citation Index   62
scientific fraud   201–3, 231
scientific meetings, paper
      presentation   241–4
search engines   32–5
   medical   35–41
SELDI-TOF   131
service-users   224
sheep models   114, 129
short-form health survey
      (SF-36)   104
slides
   35-mm   20
   paper presentation   239, 240
software packages   15, 21, 22
   see also named progams
spatial autocorrelation   190
spatial correlation   189–90
Specialist Library Guidelines
      Finder   40
specialist registrar (SpR)
   research   2
   training   1
specialist training programme   3
spellcheckers   15, 16
spellings, alternative   31
spreadsheets   18–19
   3D   19
standard deviation   155, 156
standardised mortality ratio   170
statistical analysis   109
   Bayesian analysis   161
   carrying out   155–6
   comparing proportions   157–8
   concepts   154–5
   confounding   64, 158, 160–1
   equivalence trials   101
   exploratory   155–6

methods 156–8
packages 19
planning 150
spreadsheet function 18–19
stratified 158, 160–1
thesis writing 255–6
statistical cure 185–6
statistical methods 149–50
statistical modelling,
    confounding 173–4
statistical power, clinical
    trials 105–6
statistical software 156
statistics 149–61
  disease-related 166
  distribution-free 155
  experimental design 115
  literature search 41, *43*
  non-parametric 155, 157
  official 164
  parametric 155
  sources for health-related 166
  summary 149
  see also meta-analyses
stem cells, fetal 129–30
stratification 173
  tables 158, 160–1
students 215
  expectations 218–19
  independence
      development 217–18
  needs 218–19
  project choice 215–17
  skills 216, 217
Student's *t*-test 156
study
  design 72, 73, 222–3
  population defining for clinical
      trials 102
  quality 72
subgroup analysis, clinical
    trials 106, 109
supervision 213–20
  frequency 219–20

ground rules 216–17
initial review 216
outset 215–17
periods 216
phases 220
process 214
type 219–20
supervisors
  availability 218–19
  candidate selection 215
  motivation 213–14
  project choice 215–17
  student expectations 218–19
surrogate endpoints 104, 187
surrogate tests 176
surveys 59
survival
  curves 184
  expected *185*
  observed *185*
  plot 182–3
  relative 186
survival times, censoring 182–4
syncytiotrophoblast
    preparations 129
synonyms 31
systematic reviews 59, 69
  before clinical trials 101
  sources 73–4

tables, stratified 158, 160–1
tasking 9–10
television 231
teratogenicity 128
terms, alternative 31
tests
  pathognomic 176
  performance 177
  positive predictive value 178
  results 177–8
  sensitivity/specificity 176–7, 178,
      179
  surrogate 176
therapeutic interventions 61

research design   73
thesaurus software   15
thesis writing   252–7
   computer literacy   253–4
   drafts   256
   literature reviews   254
   planning   255
   preparation   253–5
   printing   256
   production   256
   references   256
   results   255–6
   security   256
   statistical analysis   255–6
   university guidelines   255
time management   8–13
   hiding   13
   planning   8–9, 11, 223
time saving   11, 12
time series   190
time wasting   11–12
timetabling   11
tissue cultures   114
tissues, research   201
tocolytics   128
topic-based audit   85–94
training fellowships   227, 229
training programmes   2
   specialty-specific   5
   subspecialty   3
TRIP database   38, *39*
   guidelines   40
trophoblast studies   129–30
twin–twin transfusion
   syndrome   127–8
type II errors   106

UK Clinical Research Collaboration
   (UKCRC)   2
UK Ethics Committee
   Authority   197
ultrasound, fetal studies   125
unit of analysis error   109
Universities Federation for Animal
   Welfare (UFAW)   114
university guidelines   255
uterotonics   128

validation, analytic
   epidemiology   184–6
validity   64–5
variables   150–1, *152*, 155, 156
   association between   *159, 160*
   binary   157
   comparing proportions   157, 158
   correlation   158, *159*
   regression   158, *160*
vascular ablation, fetal   127
video presentations   209–10, 240
visual aids   19, 239–40
voice recognition programs   16
volunteers
   fraud elimination   203
   informed consent   199–200
vulnerable individuals   200–1

websites, appraising   35
wildcards   48, *49*
Women's Health Specialist
   Library   37, 38
word processing   15–16, 254
   integration functions   16
World Medical Assembly   195